Praise for *Has Medicine Lost Its Mind? Why Our Mental Health System Is Failing Us and What Should Be Done to Cure It*

"Somewhere along its journey through millennia, medicine lost track of the centrality of mental health in human wellness. The cost in needless suffering and avoidable death has been immense. Full of compelling patient stories and historical detail, *Has Medicine Lost Its Mind?* explains how we got here, why it matters, and what to do about it. This book is essential reading for anyone who cares about reuniting care for both the mind and the body, and anyone who has experienced the costs of failing to do so."—**Don Berwick, MD, former Administrator of the Centers for Medicare and Medicaid Services, founding president and CEO of the Institute for Healthcare Improvement, and former candidate for governor of Massachusetts**

"Mental health has long been an orphan in health care. In this timely book, Robert C. Smith argues that, now more than ever, health care needs to integrate mental and physical health. Smith shares wisdom from patients, physicians, and philosophers to remind us that splitting the mind from the body neglects both. No health without mental health has long been a refrain from mental health advocates. In this important book, Smith draws on a lifetime of experience to show us how to integrate mental and physical health to create whole-person care."—**Thomas Insel, MD, former director of the National Institute of Mental Health and author of *Healing: Our Path from Mental Illness to Mental Health***

"*Has Medicine Lost Its Mind?* tells the depressing story of our nation's failed mental health system. Like a psychoanalyst delving deep into the origin of a patient's problem, Smith explores the history beginning with mental health's infancy and the mind-body split. And as with all unresolved mental health issues, he explains how ignoring them has made their current manifestations dramatically worse. Anyone who has ever been anxious or depressed, or struggled with a family member suffering from a more serious psychological problem, will find comfort in the solutions he proposes."—**Dr. Robert Pearl, professor at Stanford University Business and Medical School and author of *Uncaring: How the Culture of Medicine Kills Doctors and Patients* and *ChatGPT, MD: How AI-Empowered Patients and Doctors Can Take Back Control of American Medicine***

"A passionate plea for reforming medical education from a doctor who has devoted his career to teaching student doctors how to listen to patients. Robert C. Smith now he goes on to describe the benefits that would flow if all physicians knew how to understand and help mental health problems. Patients would benefit, of course, but his proposal could also improve physician satisfaction and medicine as a whole."—**Randolph Nesse, professor emeritus of psychiatry at the University of Michigan, a founder of the field of evolutionary medicine, and author of** *Good Reasons for Bad Feelings: Insights from the Frontier of Evolutionary Psychiatry*

"The answer is a convincing 'yes,' medicine has lost its mind. But there is hope! Using data from important clinical studies and remarkable stories from his practice, Smith lays out the lament, a call to action, and a path to progress. This is an important and thought-provoking assessment and plan for anyone interested in how our mental health crisis became so bad and how we can solve it."—**Aron Sousa, MD, FACP, Dean, College of Human Medicine, Michigan State University**

"This book offers a comprehensive understanding of the staggering neglect of the mental well-being of our nation's people and an equally comprehensive prescription for solving this shortfall. Like a good systems thinker, Robert C. Smith ties it all together, from training to policymaking, from conversing with patients to adopting new paradigms of health. Smith brings to bear formidable knowledge, wisdom, and judgment, fifty years in the making, and offers us a coherent way forward—as citizens, patients, activists, clinicians, educators, and policymakers. I recommend this timely book to anyone who cares about the future of medicine, health care, or the health of the people in this nation."—**Frank deGruy, MD, MSFM, distinguished professor in the Department of Family Medicine at the University of Colorado School of Medicine**

"In this compelling book, Robert C. Smith, an internist and prominent figure in biopsychosocial medicine, advocates for transformative reform in the health care system. He emphasizes the need to integrate biopsychosocial principles into patient care to revive the true spirit of medicine. Smith shares his experiences and challenges during his medical training, which highlight the emotional consequences of feeling that he provided inadequate support for his patients, prompting him to rethink his approach to care. This thoughtful and well-written book will help readers understand the current health care crisis and the need for federal intervention to correct it."—**Douglas A. Drossman, MD, professor emeritus of medicine and psychiatry at the University of North Carolina at Chapel Hill and CEO and president emeritus of the Rome Foundation**

Has Medicine Lost Its Mind?

Why Our Mental Health System Is Failing Us and What Should Be Done to Cure It

ROBERT C. SMITH, MD

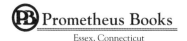
Prometheus Books

Essex, Connecticut

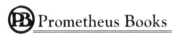 Prometheus Books

An imprint of The Globe Pequot Publishing Group, Inc.
64 South Main Street
Essex, CT 06426
www.globepequot.com

Distributed by NATIONAL BOOK NETWORK

British Library Cataloguing in Publication Information Available

Library of Congress Cataloging-in-Publication Data Available

ISBN 9781493087655 (cloth : alk. paper) | ISBN 9781493087662 (epub)

∞™ The paper used in this publication meets the minimum requirements of American National Standard for Information Sciences—Permanence of Paper for Printed Library Materials, ANSI/NISO Z39.48-1992.

The information in this book should not be construed as a recommendation for treatment. Those with mental health problems should consult their care providers.

ALSO BY ROBERT C. SMITH

Smith's Patient-Centered Interviewing: An Evidence-Based Method

Essentials of Psychiatry in Primary Care: Behavioral Health in the Medical Setting

For my wife, Susan Sleeper-Smith—
my guide, my friend, and the love of my life.

Contents

Part I

THE MENTAL HEALTH CARE PROBLEM

CHAPTER 1

US Mental Health Care Breaks Down

Medicine is losing its soul by dismissing mental health care and other psychological and social dimensions of its patients and by ignoring the very features that make us human. I believe we must improve mental health care and that we can revive medicine's spirit and soul in so doing. (Except where noted, the book uses the terms *mental* and *psychological* to include substance-use problems.)

Why should you be concerned? Mental health difficulties in one way or another have almost certainly touched you and your loved ones because of how common these problems have become. Mental disorders are the most common health condition that physicians face in daily practice, far exceeding the combined numbers of patients with heart disease and cancer, according to the National Alliance for Mental Illness.[1] Research from the National Institute of Mental Health projects that one-half of the entire US population will experience a mental disorder at some point during their lives and that, in any given year, one-fourth of Americans will have a major mental illness.[2] In other words, roughly every family of four will, on average, have one member with a mental disorder this coming year.[3] Two recent studies provide the exact numbers: The 2020 National Survey on Drug Use and Health indicates that 39.7 million people had a substance-abuse problem of some type (alcohol, illicit drugs); the National Alliance on Mental Illness indicates that there were 52.9 million persons with a mental illness unrelated to drug abuse in 2020.[4] Combine the two and you have *more than 90 million people with a significant mental disorder in 2020.*

In the same year, less than half of patients with a mental disorder and less than 10 percent with a substance-use problem had any access to care.[5] In another study from the Department of Health and Human Services (DHHS), only 25 percent of patients with mental illnesses in the United States have any access to care because there is so little help available. This means that three-fourths of patients with a major mental disorder do not receive care.[6] Research from Harvard Medical School generated similar findings when they demon-strated that fewer than one-third of patients with a major mental disorder received care.[7] Compare these low statistics to the whopping 60–80 percent of patients with a physical disease who do receive care, according to the Depart-ment of Health and Human Services.[8]

Three values steer present-day medicine: quality of care, access to care, and safety of care. While the medical establishment embraces this triumvirate of principles, it employs them only for physical illnesses and largely ignores them when it comes to patients with mental health issues—and other psychological and social issues, as well.

Untreated mental illnesses devastate the American population. I know this from my own family's various problems. If you've not had personal experiences, you almost certainly have learned from the internet, newspapers, and television of society's many tragic deaths from suicides and overdoses.[9] These tragedies permeate the fabric of our society. Far more people end up so disabled with psychological issues—such as depression, anxiety, or substance abuse—that they cannot, for example, go to church, attend movies, play golf, go shopping, visit grandchildren, or even have sex. Sadly, I've seen many of these difficulties mush-room into more serious complications, such as strained relationships, divorce, job loss, school failure, substance abuse, legal hot water, and even incarceration and homelessness.[10] I give lots of case examples later.

To the chagrin of taxpayers, the ramifications of poor or no mental health care extend well beyond individual patients because they afflict society with ex-cessive health care costs. *Has Medicine Lost Its Mind?* shows how the American health care system could significantly improve patients' health while simultane-ously reducing our nation's overall health care budget by trillions of dollars. Yes, I know that's a bold statement, but stick with me, and you'll see how.

If these overlooked problems leave you flabbergasted, then *Has Medicine Lost Its Mind?* is here to help. It is a clarion call to activate the public to instigate change in the way the health care system and the medical profession deal with mental health problems—and reclaim medicine's soul along the way. Today's medical profession governs itself, and it fails Americans in their psychological health. Even more troublesome, it has evinced little interest in adjusting its course. Only an informed public and its politicians can prompt change in the status quo.

In the final chapter, *Has Medicine Lost Its Mind?* describes the specific po-litical mechanism to disrupt the status quo. Then, appendixes B and C describe exactly what to do.

———◆———

As an internal medicine physician, I went into the profession to help people and to allay suffering. The following guidance from Hippocrates meant something to me: "Cure sometimes, treat often, comfort always" and "*Primum non nocere*," meaning "First, do no harm."[11]

But I have not always lived up to my Hippocratic oath. Despite my role as an internist and my concerns regarding mental illness, I, like so many other doctors, personified the mental health care predicament. For more than half my patients—those with a psychological illness—I did not cure, did not treat, and did not comfort.

Seeing such patients during my medical school and subsequent residency education made me feel like an abject failure—a feeling that only became more pressing when I entered practice and faced many more mental health issues. Fellow colleagues told me of similar worries when we talked over a beer or two. The medical education we had spent years undergoing had not prepared us. It lacked even rudimentary preparation for dealing with mental illness. In practice, we flew by the seat of our pants when we tried to help this large patient population.

During our medical education, we trained under kind, decent physicians. But, though they cared about their patients, they had little time for emotions or psychological issues. As students and residents, we followed suit. From many conversations with fellow learners, I recognized that, down deep, our patients' mental disorders and other personal difficulties troubled many of us, but we didn't know what to do or say—and generally did nothing at all.

SVEN'S STORY

One patient from my residency troubles me to this day. Sven entered the hospital with high blood pressure, and it proved uncontrollable over the months to follow. Sven was fifty years old, an outgoing, kind man who suffered from severe, debilitating headaches. His blood pressure was as high as 230/135 when we admitted him to the university hospital where I trained—so high it had already damaged his eyes (where he had small hemorrhages and narrowed blood vessels at the back [the retina] of his eyes); his kidneys (where he had blood and protein in his urine); and his heart (which was enlarged). He was always upbeat, and I liked him and his slightly off-color jokes: "Have you heard the one about . . . ?" I was personally devastated with what followed over the next several months.

I left that teaching rotation after a month. When I returned two months later, he was still in the hospital, but his vivacity had vanished. Now, curled up in the far corner of his bed, he answered questions in monosyllables. I cringed at what had happened to him. His blood pressure was lower but still too high, and his kidneys and heart were deteriorating. He died four months after admission.

Sadly, no one ever talked to Sven about the personal impact of his illness. No one even broached the idea of depression, nor did I or anyone proffer emotional support. I felt paralyzed, not knowing how to help or whether I should even address personal issues. I wondered why our faculty did nothing. I could tell by the worry I saw on their faces that they cared, but their attitude conveyed hopelessness. We simply had nothing else to offer but attending to his physical disease.

Hauntingly, I remember the brightly colored toothpaste tube on Sven's bedside stand: Vademecum. With peculiar staying power, it still shines brightly today in my mind's eye. After his death, I happened on the Latin phrase *vade mecum* in the dictionary.[12] It instantly brought back the angst I felt about Sven's illness when I learned its original meaning: "Go with me." I hadn't gone with him. No one did. We deserted him—in his time of greatest need—as my colleagues and I lost part of our souls.

Today, far more powerful medications probably would control Sven's blood pressure. He had an uncommon form of hypertension called malignant hypertension—"malignant" because its rapid progression to death resembles some particularly severe cancers. But today, not much has changed in providing care for how patients psychologically deal with a bad disease. A plight similar to Sven's befalls the millions of patients with advanced, severe illnesses, like cancer, heart disease, emphysema, or Alzheimer's disease, that lead to death or severe disability. Medicine still avoids these patients' pressing personal needs, as we did with Sven.

No one ever considered offering Sven a psychiatric consultation. This type of help took place far from the main hospital, where, as everyone called them, the "crazy" patients received care. Not always in jest, we often said the psychiatrists had troubles similar to their patients. This negative attitude was commonly displayed toward psychiatry and mental issues, which persists today.

I had no perception of what I was facing when I went into medical practice. My blithely unaware, overconfident attitude would soon shatter. The experience I disclose here—with reservation and guilt even today—represents only the worst of many. Though painful, this occurrence opened my eyes and slowly but unalterably transformed my life.

APRIL'S STORY

April was new to the city, forty years old. A prominent physician in another city had referred her to my senior internist partner. Our group of six doctors provided primary care and consulted with other clinicians on difficult cases. When my busy partner could not accept her, she came to me. April's transfer note explained that she had metastatic breast cancer, which had spread to her lower spine, causing considerable pain. She had received all the chemotherapy and radiation available at the time. No other treatment remained. The referral note indicated her doctor had told her this but that she still didn't seem to understand her dire outlook. I was new in practice, thirty-one years old.

When I first met April, I reacted in two ways: I liked her sophisticated, intellectual style and her attractive appearance, but my anxiety and fear soon overshadowed these and, mirroring hers, came to dominate our interactions.

April was often semifrantic and wanted to know our plan of action. "How do I get well?" she always asked, but I knew I had nothing to offer. She was not demanding, even somewhat passive and deferential, and I felt sorry for her. But I had no idea how to help her. At various visits, she implored, "Can't you do something? I'm so out of hope. Why am I getting worse? I can't sleep. My life seems no fun. Why do I cry all the time?" Feeling guilty and inadequate, I would order another X-ray or some other test, even though I knew I conveyed the false hope that something good might come of it. At least it bought time—for me. April's husband never came with her, but I would encounter him at the time of her death. I didn't ask April about him or her support for what must have been her severe depression.

But when she steadied and calmed down at various times, so did I. We then had some good, less-tense moments. She and I talked about her kids and how she took them to music camp each summer. Fluent in French, she loved everything about the culture. Still, I avoided discussing the expected outcome of her cancer. To do so scared me. Even when she alluded to it, I'd say something noncommittal like, "We'll just have to see."

I felt like a failure, powerless. I dreaded her visits. Each new or altered symptom frightened April, and rather than talk by phone, she wanted me to see her—for the pain, her inability to eat or sleep, her weight loss, her constipation from the narcotics, and her increasing view that her life was "no fun." And she had an ever-constant question: "What do I do? Can't you help?" She always gave me a haunting, wan smile as she left my office.

As I expected, April progressively worsened and eventually died. In her final hospital stay, I was surprised to see her husband, children, and so many others who cared about her. Until that moment, I had seen her alone, struggling to survive, as if she existed solely in the exam room or the hospital bed.

I felt bad for April and the family. Despite all our turmoil, I had gotten to know her and liked her. But I would not miss her and her constant, impossible questions. Mostly, I felt relief from my feelings of guilt and inadequacy. Until a few weeks later.

Her husband arrived unannounced at my office and asked to see me. In going through her private belongings after she died, he had found a diary she kept and thought it would interest me. He left quickly, a hurried exit that made me uneasy. I soon learned why he slipped out so fast.

April's journal contained many comments about my care: "Now that there's no other treatment, the young doctor doesn't seem to know what to do with me. . . . He just orders more tests. . . . So depressed, so alone. . . . Why doesn't he understand? . . . That would help. . . . I don't think he cares."

After reading many similar entries, I stopped, unable to continue. I thought, "My God, I'm a doctor, and I did not even try to help this anguished, tormented human being I cared about. What about April's comfort and peace of mind? Aren't I responsible for taking care of those? What about the Hippocratic Oath?"

That morning, I felt increasingly troubled and restive. And my stomach gnawed furiously, something new to me. I couldn't concentrate. My thoughts wandered while seeing other patients, continually returning to April's diary—and her plaintive face. The scribbles from her feeble hand, her mournful look. I couldn't shake them. They intruded uncontrollably over the next several weeks. An unsettling inner turmoil lasted much longer; indeed, pangs of guilt and a sense of wrongdoing reawaken as I write about this now, decades later. Shaken to my very core, I slowly resolved to turn over a new leaf. The only thing I knew to change at this point was to consciously listen and respond to what patients were saying and to hear their problems even if they involved nonmedical issues—and to avoid interrupting to ask medical questions.

Going forward, I began to understand patients better, but my progress evolved ever so slowly. Patients with different types of psychological issues, especially chronic pain, challenged me, and there were many of them because of the nature of my practice. As I mentioned, I was an internist, part of a six-physician practice to whom other doctors referred difficult patients. This was a time when few specialists were available, and because I was well-trained in a university hospital, the many family medicine practitioners in the area welcomed me for consultations with difficult patients. I also had a primary care practice. I received referrals for a variety of medical issues, such as weight loss, difficult-to-manage diabetes, refractory asthma, unexplained fevers, and bleeding from the bowels.

These referrals also included many challenging patients with long-standing unexplained pain in locations varying from the low back to the neck to headaches. Of course, the referring doctors and their patients wanted to know the disease diagnosis and treatment, so I would perform an extensive examination along with many X-rays and other tests. I seldom found a disease explanation for the pain. At first, I would happily and naively tell patients, "Good news, there's nothing wrong."

This diagnosis was not well received. "You mean this is all in my head? Do you think I'm making this up?" They wanted answers but not one with psychological implications, which they understood as an insult. Early on, after giving one patient such "good news," I got a call from the man's referring doctor, who chided me, "He's angrier at you than me now. I guess you were some help!" I was afraid to ask but secretly wondered how he and other physicians handled these problems. I didn't know how.

I'd never seen such angry and depressed patients in my training, and as with April and Sven, I initially fared badly in relieving their discomfort. But in time, as I slowly began to realize that they agonized considerably and not just from their pain, I began to listen and commiserate—and grow. The pain affected their life situations, bringing on joblessness; relationship disruptions; and, understandably, feelings of depression, anger, and hopelessness. Several patients even commented how it helped to have someone listen and understand.

After a while, as I listened more, I noticed that many pain patients told me about difficult family circumstances, so I began seeing them regularly to talk. To my great surprise, some got better. For example, I said to one man, "You told me the headaches began when your mother-in-law moved in with you?" Well, the bitter, expletive-laced tirade that ensued that morning cannot be printed, but over many visits, this man improved. No, he didn't evict his mother-in-law. Rather, our direct engagement—the act of our talking and my understanding him—fostered improvement. I helped my patients, while they helped me learn.

Fast-forward several years. My increasing openness to patients clearly benefited them. And to my surprise, I realized that it felt good getting to know them. I no longer felt so hurried. In fact, I secretly relished our talks. Why secretly? Our professors had drummed into us, "Keep your distance. Patients don't want to talk about touchy-feely things." Others admonished, "Don't get personal. It will interfere with being objective."

JOAN'S STORY

Now, when an opportunity arose to try to relieve a patient's severe misery—similar to Sven's and April's—I embraced it but always with uncertainty; I still didn't know anything about mental health, even though I'd learned to listen more attentively. Terminal patients were among my most troubling. One patient, Joan, had an advanced lymphoma (lymph-node cancer) in her neck. All possible treatment had been exhausted. Her husband had left her some time before, which prompted her to move back to her hometown, where I practiced. She first came to me about a year before she died with complications caused by the surgery and radiation she received, which had irremediably damaged her vocal cords. It left her with a raspy, grating voice and an open wound near her larynx (voice box) that would not heal. Pus oozed continuously, leading her to avoid social interactions. She had no appetite, and antibiotics provided only brief help. She couldn't work, and large doses of antidepressant medications held only meager relief for her severe depression. She had repeatedly refused to see a mental health professional. Her life was miserable. I was at wit's end and didn't know what to do. But I felt terrible for her and listened sympathetically to her complaints.

We talked at length over several months about her quandary, mostly regarding her feelings of despair and the incredible difficulty of everyday life. She no longer wanted to live this way. She finally asked, "Can you help? I just can't continue. I don't want to. You've been so good to me." I was more torn than ever, but in a tearful session at her hospital bedside, along with the young nurse who worked closely with us over Joan's many hospital admissions, the three of us discussed Joan's suggested strategy. For the first time since I'd known her, she smiled and hugged me. Joan died peacefully the next morning; she had escaped the misery of her daily existence.

Although I made progress in supporting patients emotionally and often helped them with my empathy and caring, I could see I had still further to go. I still saw chronic pain patients I couldn't help. Even sending them to specialists did no good. I was frustrated and puzzled. And the alcohol problems of so many disturbed me and seemed just as difficult to treat. For example, I saw a patient I faintly knew from playing tennis at the same facility; I'll call him Steve. After examining him and doing some tests, I told him that he had to stop drinking because he had an enlarged liver and the blood tests showed major damage. Steve was to come back in a week, and we'd work on a plan. He returned on schedule but was still drinking a lot. Oddly to me, Steve gave me an expensive wristwatch as a gift. I, of course, refused and reiterated we needed to work together to stop drinking. We set some plans for how to cut down, and he was to see me regularly so we could try some medications. I never saw him again. I then learned some eighteen months later that he died of liver failure. Terribly chagrined, I asked myself, "What did I do wrong?"

Furthermore, I didn't know how to adequately diagnose mental illnesses. And the medications for them baffled me, especially for managing patients with depression or those whose frightening panic attacks often brought them to the emergency room with chest pain. Clearly, I needed to do more than listen. Indeed, the more I learned about my patients' personal issues, the more troubled I became, because I still didn't have sufficient knowledge to ease their burden.

While I had learned much from my practice partners, I made the difficult decision to leave my practice in order to develop better skills in mental health and the other psychological and social aspects of medicine. Uncertain of my future and how to finance this change was scary, but things seemed to just fall into place. During my last year in practice, I learned of the Los Angeles Center for the Healing Arts and was invited to work there for one year; I could support myself by emergency-room work at a large city hospital. Also, during the year before leaving practice, I contacted my chief of medicine from my residency days to seek input on how best to establish a career in the psychological and social aspects of medicine. He knew immediately what I was talking about and put me in touch with the University of Rochester and its Medical-Psychiatric Liaison Program led by Dr. George Engel.

I'd never heard of the program or Dr. Engel, but it was to become one of the greatest gifts of my life. I still recall the fateful evening when, following some introductory correspondence in the weeks beforehand, Dr. Engel called and invited me to join their two-year fellowship program after my year in Los Angeles. Dr. Engel would become a friend and mentor with a powerful impact on my life and career. It was under his tutelage that I garnered the confidence needed to pursue an academic career. I would remain in close touch with him until his death in 1999.

Amazed at how everything had fallen into place, I was not disappointed. My year at the Los Angeles Center for the Healing Arts provided me with a rich background in meditation, learning about myself, and some alternative approaches to medicine. The following year, I moved to Rochester, New York, for what would become the defining period of my professional life. The training would fill the many gaps in my knowledge and skill base, especially communicating effectively, establishing a doctor-patient relationship, and addressing mental disorders.

It was not easy by any means. In fact, much of my new learning was quite different from anything I'd experienced before. But the faculty and other fellows provided just the support I needed. Indeed, that was one of my first learnings: the importance in teaching about the teacher-learner relationship.

And I became exposed for the first time to the patient-centered interview and its centrality to learning about patients' most meaningful psychological and social concerns, which, in turn, established strong relationships. You'll hear much about this later in the book, including how to conduct it. It was not easy to learn for control-oriented physicians like me because it requires new skills and relinquishing some control to the patient.

In yet another new learning experience, the fellowship program offered psychoanalytic therapy if the fellow chose to participate. I eagerly took this opportunity to better understand myself. It proved crucial not only personally but also for addressing patients' psychological, emotional, and social issues. They can easily trip one's own emotional responses and alter the effectiveness of treatment and the relationship. For example, before I recognized my need to control, seeing a controlling patient often prompted me to compete for control—not a good thing for our relationship! Nor was this learning easy. It came only with time and a patient, caring teacher. I have come to agree with those who believe that psychotherapy for clinicians is essential if they plan to work with patients' mental health and other personal issues.

Another new experience was learning about the lives of patients with severe mental disorders, from my psychotic inpatient who saw me as her brother to the teenager who carried an ax about his house, demolishing furniture. One patient I cared for became psychotic, during our clinical work, because of chronic pain and her loss of an infant. My less severe, primary care patients were not any easier. For example, I had to learn the hard way that some patients did not want me to do specific things to help them. Rather, they just wanted to be listened to and supported. Learning the myriad medications the doctor could use and conducting psychotherapy required additional time and careful supervision from my teachers.

And finally, there was my intellectually stimulating learning about the theoretical basis for a new medicine. Dr. Engel had articulated the general systems–based biopsychosocial model shortly before I matriculated at Rochester.[13] Seeing my conceptual interest, he provided extensive reading material and spent considerable personal time teaching me the nuances and details of general systems theory. You'll hear much more about the biopsychosocial model later in this book and the central role of Dr. Engel in the new science of medicine. This new model would become my guiding principle in articulating Engel's view of medicine that enhances not only the science but also the humanity of medicine—its soul.

As a result of my learning, I developed considerable empathy for the uphill battle the untrained primary care clinician would have to overcome to succeed in mental health care. It's way too complex for on-the-job training while in full-time practice. This realization led me to commit my career to teaching primary care mental health while future practitioners were still in training. This direction was further enriched when I began working with many like-minded national and international colleagues in an organization now called the Academy of Communication in Healthcare—an organization devoted, as the name suggests, to improving the communication of physicians and other health care professionals with patients. These experiences not only fostered my professional development and teaching skills but also my personal growth.

I left Rochester after six years, the last four on faculty, a much-changed man, more confident in addressing the psychological and social dimensions of medicine. I was thankful for the many mentors and friends who had been so helpful. I resolved to improve primary care mental health via research and teaching.

After a brief stint at St. Louis University, where I learned much about chronic pain and the nuances of its management, I moved to Michigan State University, where my career would unfold over the next nearly forty years. Already well versed in the biopsychosocial model and with much expertise in primary care and patient-based care, this community-based medical school fit my interests perfectly. And it had another attribute that met my needs: openness to new ideas, to fostering a different direction. For example, when I would identify a teaching or research problem I wanted to work on, I was at first surprised to hear them say, "Why not? How can we help?" To cite just one example, I wanted to teach residents psychosocial medicine and patient-centered interviewing in a one-month, full-time block. Of course, all the monthly blocks were already taken. No problem. My division chief and residency director creatively worked out a new scheduling system: They converted from a twelve-month schedule to a thirteen-month (lunar) schedule and gave me the new month. They never stopped saying, "Why not?" and providing the support to facilitate my work.

In this propitious Michigan State atmosphere, I found the many scholars—from the disciplines of medicine, family medicine, ethics, psychiatry, epidemiology, radiology, medical education, physiology, communication, and linguistics—who became crucial to my continued growth and understanding as an educator and researcher. And I was especially fortunate to have great external consultants looking over my shoulder on many research projects, as well as to receive support from several federal and private granting agencies.

My Michigan State career began in patient-centered interviewing, and, incorporating interviewing as the first step, it soon morphed into primary care mental health—with extensive research in both areas. As the basis for much of this activity, I was fortunate to have the opportunity to teach students, especially residents. My research on teaching residents established the first evidence-based teaching model for patient-centered interviewing and, later, the first one for primary care mental health care.[14] Our textbook describing the interviewing model, *Smith's Patient-Centered Interviewing: An Evidence-Based Method*, is now widely used for teaching students, residents, and practitioners of medicine, nursing, and allied professions.[15] Also designed for teaching this same group of learners, the mental health care model is described in our new psychiatry textbook, *Essentials of Psychiatry in Primary Care: Behavioral Health in the Medical Setting*.[16]

It's been a true odyssey to have come full circle to help future primary care clinicians effectively address mental health issues. While my textbooks describe how individual teachers and clinicians can do this, *Has Medicine Lost Its Mind?* articulates the path for implementing better mental health care on a national scale by challenging the status quo to make a true paradigm shift—and restore medicine's soul along the way.

CHAPTER 2

The Cause of Poor Mental Health Care

It has long been recognized that there is an extreme shortage of mental health care professionals in the United States. This has led to the stunning fact that *most treatment of mental health problems is conducted by primary care and other medical physicians who are not trained to diagnose and treat mental disorders.* Yet those in charge of health care planning continue to omit this training in the medical schools and residencies that prepare physicians for clinical practice. The result: substandard care for most with mental illnesses like depression and, more broadly, those with less severe but very common mental health issues, such as stress. Medicine does not live up to the high principles it embraces—ease of access to care, quality of care, and safety of care.

How has the health care planning process gone so awry? Who can society identify as being responsible for the current situation? The planners for medical-student education are a large, diverse group of medical school deans and educators and their national governing body, the Association of American Medical Colleges; for residency education, they are multiple program directors and their national governing agency, the Accreditation Council for Graduate Medical Education. These groups determine what represents sufficient training of medical students and residents to ensure quality health care for American citizens.

To be fair, organizing medicine to produce treatment of actual diseases is not haphazard. Who can forget the immediate response to the Zika virus when epidemiology researchers discovered that the deadly virus, spread by mosquitos, had reached epidemic levels in Brazil and rapidly spread through the rest of South America? Congress appropriated $1.1 billion to control and curtail the disease.[1] The profession has launched similar successful public health wars against cancer, heart disease, and COVID-19.[2] In short, those who organize our health care have successfully developed strategies to deal with the physical disorders of every organ and body element—from hair loss on our heads to bunions and fungal infections of our feet.

But when it comes to mental disorders, medicine all too often falls silent, leaving clinicians to cope by themselves—or not. In most instances, clinicians overlook the mental condition. Or if they happen to recognize the problem, they often stigmatize the patient for being mentally ill, as reported in a 2016 study by the National Academies of Sciences, Engineering, and Medicine.[3]

Mental Health Professionals: Insufficient Numbers for Society's Needs

If medicine and its architects had a strategy for comprehensive psychological care for all Americans, then one might guess they would name mental health specialists as its centerpiece. However, the grossly deficient numbers of mental health practitioners preclude them as the solution to effective care for most of the population. Compounding this shortfall in numbers, the United States has seen an increased demand for mental health care due to three factors: the population's growth; the fact that many more people have health insurance because of the Affordable Care Act; and, most recently, the COVID-19 pandemic.[4]

The Health Resources and Services Administration reports that in 2017 our frontline mental health workforce comprised the following: 91,440 psychologists; 33,650 adult psychiatrists; 8,090 child and adolescent psychiatrists; 10,450 psychiatric nurse practitioners; and 1,550 psychiatric physician assistants.[5] These professionals receive the extensive education required to serve as the primary caretakers for all levels of mental illness severity, from psychosis on one extreme to daily stress on the other. Psychologists primarily conduct outpatient psychotherapy and counseling. Psychiatrists provide hospital care for severe disorders, such as schizophrenia, as well as conduct outpatient practices, usually limited to medication management. Several additional mental health specialists—although not taught comprehensive psychological care—play more restricted but still crucial roles, as their names indicate, such as social workers, family and marriage therapists, and licensed counselors for addiction and schools.

To see how this shortage plays out in real terms, I first look at psychiatrists. Psychiatrists see but a small fraction of all patients with mental disorders, only 12.3 percent, according to research from the National Institute of Mental Health.[6] Do psychiatrists care for so few patients because they spend so much time with each one?[7] No, the old fifty-minute hour vanished with the advent of ten- to fifteen-minute visits focused on medications. Scarcely 10 percent of psychiatrists practice psychotherapy today.[8] With such short visits, then, why the problem? Insufficient numbers both now and in the past explain it. Compounding the supply shortage, experts project the total number of psychiatrists to fall from 41,740 (combined adult and child psychiatrists) to 38,821 by 2024 and to 36,850 by 2030.[9]

The shortage surprises no one. A review identified it during a study of the years 1974–1981.[10] And the General Medical Education National Advisory Committee formally predicted it more than three decades ago.[11] How bad is it? So few psychiatrists now practice in America that two-thirds of primary care doctors cannot obtain even a consultation for a troubled patient.[12] Experts judge that more than 95 percent of US counties have insufficient numbers of practicing psychiatrists; 50 percent of rural counties have no psychiatrists at all.[13] Intensifying the shortage, psychiatrists—and psychologists—tend to locate in affluent urban areas and university towns, especially in the Northeast, a practice unaltered since 1978.[14] Meanwhile, from 2003 to 2013, the number of psychiatry residencies and its graduates—the source of future psychiatrists—declined overall.[15]

Yet, as I mentioned in chapter 1, more than 90 million Americans will experience one or more major mental disorders in any given year, each needing multiple visits and detailed attention.[16] If the psychiatric workforce furnished care for all these patients, then the minimum number of patients per psychiatrist would exceed two thousand. And these data do not include the far greater numbers of patients with less-severe mental health difficulties. Although data are scarce, surveys estimate that psychiatrists now have average caseloads of about two hundred to three hundred, seeing an average of around twelve patients per day.[17]

Why this dearth of psychiatrists? Some startling research from the *British Journal of Psychiatry* suggests that something happens during medical school to alter students' views of psychiatry.[18] This study found that, among those entering medical school, 49 percent express significant interest in psychiatry. However, when graduating four years later, only 4 percent choose to specialize in this field. This loss of interest during four years of teaching demands an explanation.[19] Something happens during this time to alter students' views of psychiatry.

It is possible that students' limited exposure to mental illness during medical school could be to blame, or perhaps it's due to the fact that financial compensation for psychiatrists is low.[20] But I and others propose a deeper, more fundamental issue—that a harmful culture of medicine exists, one that values the body and its diseases but diminishes mind-related and psychosocial issues, sometimes actually disdaining them.[21] Students repeatedly experience these damaging attitudes in their interactions with faculty over four years of education and convert to an antipsychiatry mindset. You will hear much more about medicine's pernicious culture later in the book.

Now let us look at the situation with psychologists. More than twice as many psychologists as psychiatrists care for patients, providing 16 percent of all mental health care, so this improves the situation slightly—but still not nearly enough to serve the population nationwide.[22] Although data are in short supply, psychologists often conduct psychotherapy for thirty to sixty minutes per patient, in contrast to ten- to fifteen-minute visits by psychiatrists. This suggests they work with smaller caseloads of patients than psychiatrists—a fact that could mitigate the effect of their greater numbers.

Surprisingly, some question the role of psychology in caring for mental health problems and worry that psychologists lack expertise in prescribing medications and providing care in clinics or hospital settings where patients have coexisting medical disorders. These two concerns do not at all hold up on closer examination, in my opinion, nor should they obscure the role for psychology as part of a solution to limited mental health care.[23] Regarding the first issue, research demonstrates that psychologists perform psychotherapy that can actually match or exceed the effectiveness of drug prescriptions for depression and anxiety. At the same time, patients often prefer therapy to medications.[24] This offsets the possible drawback of their inability to prescribe. Plus, policies evolve; five states now allow psychologists to prescribe medications if they participate in additional education.[25] As for the second concern—ability to administer care in medical settings—in 2014, the American Psychological Association advocated greatly increased training in clinics and hospitals, published a set of competencies psychologists should possess, and urged its PhD graduates to acquire the skills for working with patients in medical settings so they can better integrate psychological issues with physical disease difficulties.[26] I have personally worked with the first group to conduct this training—in Flint, Michigan—and can attest to its production of highly skilled clinicians fit for medical settings.[27]

In sum, given the even smaller numbers of physician assistants and nurse practitioners skilled in mental health care, the numbers of trained mental health providers capable of giving comprehensive, frontline care do not even come close to meeting the need. Because of this, mental health professionals have had little impact on care from a population perspective. In my opinion, medicine must educate more psychologists, psychiatrists, psychiatric nurse practitioners, and psychiatric physician assistants. Indeed, I advocate this as part of my proposal for improved patient care, which I explain later.

Primary Care and Other Physicians: Unqualified in Mental Health

While studies vary slightly, primary care doctors (in general practice, family medicine, internal medicine, pediatrics, obstetrics/gynecology) and, to a far lesser degree, other more specialized practitioners (such as surgery or dermatology) conduct care for about 75 percent of Americans with mental illnesses, even though they lack appropriate training.[28] And it's not just the scarcity of mental health professionals. Just as significant is that the average individual usually consults his or her primary care physician first with any health difficulties, whether psychological or physical.

That there is a significantly greater number of medical physicians than mental health professionals suggests that they could well be the solution for handling mental health difficulties—but they would need to be trained. Primary care and other physicians are far more widely distributed across the United States and carry much larger numbers of patients in their practices. In 2020, the Kaiser Family Foundation reported that there were 1,022,006 total active MD and DO practitioners, of which there were 486,405 in primary care and 535,601 specialists.[29] The average number of patients in a primary care practice just exceeded 2,300 patients.[30]

Given the shortage of mental health experts, you'd expect that savvy organizers would see to it that medical schools train all physicians in mental health care, especially those planning primary care practices, to ensure they graduate as competent in treating mental disorders as they are in treating medical disorders. Yet the Association of American Medical Colleges, the organization charged with setting curricula for all medical schools offering an MD, tells us that, despite thousands of hours of medical education devoted to organic diseases, medical students receive on average only 5.1 weeks of psychiatry training. Out of four years of medical education, this is their only supervised clinical experience with mental illnesses.[31]

Look at an average medical school curriculum to fully appreciate this disparity. Each of the following experiences lasts several weeks to months. Scanning the list of topics, you'll note an almost exclusive interest in bodily issues and physical diseases; the few exposures concerning mental health and other psychosocial issues are in italics:

- **Preclinical Curriculum (Years 1 and 2):** Of a total of 1,463 hours of required teaching, behavioral sciences receive 56 hours (3.8 percent):[32]

    Year 1: anatomy, histology, physiology, biochemistry, genetics, epidemiology, neuroscience, clinical skills, *behavioral sciences*
    Year 2: pathology, microbiology, parasitology, pharmacology, clinical skills, statistics, *behavioral sciences*

- **Clinical Curriculum (Years 3 and 4):** Except for 5.1 weeks of psychiatry in year 3 (less than 5 percent of total time), all are primarily, if not exclusively, devoted to the physical diseases addressed by each discipline:[33]

Year 3: family medicine (some provide a modicum of *psychiatry*); internal medicine; obstetrics/gynecology; pediatrics; surgery; neurology; allergy/immunology; surgical subspecialties (orthopedics, ophthalmology, otolaryngology, urology, neurosurgery); radiology; electives; *psychiatry*

Year 4: family medicine (some provide a modicum of *psychiatry*); internal medicine; obstetrics/gynecology; pediatrics; surgery; neurology; allergy/immunology; surgical subspecialties (orthopedics, ophthalmology, otolaryngology, urology, neurosurgery); radiology; electives (less than 5 percent choose an elective in *psychiatry*)

What's the impact of lack of training? Medical clinicians typically falter in recognizing mental disorders, much less advance effective treatment or refer patients for counseling, according to research from my group at Michigan State.[34] Additionally, multiple researchers have demonstrated that, when clinicians do attempt to provide care, it usually does not meet standards, further jeopardizing both quality and safety of care.[35] For example, Harvard Medical School researchers found that doctors often prescribe mental health medications for the wrong conditions, and when they do prescribe the correct drug for a mental disorder, they seldom recommend the effective dose or advise follow-up.[36] Other researchers observed the same problem: 60 to 70 percent of mental health patients seen in medical settings receive no treatment whatsoever; when clinicians do prescribe, it fails nearly 90 percent of the time.[37] It comes as no surprise that researchers find primary care clinicians have low levels of comfort in treating psychiatric conditions.[38]

Does it strike you as bizarre that the medical profession does not teach doctors to treat half of the patients they will see in practice? If other professions acted similarly, then lawyers might only understand the plaintiff role, dentists might only know how to pull teeth, and universities might only teach the humanities.

Given the current mental health crisis—the crisis in access, quality, and safety of care I've described—one would expect planning experts to mandate that residencies conduct mental health care education. (Residency follows medical school as the last formal training for many physicians before they enter practice.) Unfortunately, they don't. Residencies deliver even less instruction in mental disorders than medical schools do; most offer none at all.[39] While family medicine residencies do better than other primary care residencies, I'm embarrassed to say that internal medicine devotes a median of only seventeen hours per year to its mental health curriculum—one or two lunchtime lectures each month.[40] But meaningful training requires much more time and supervision with actual patients. Further, the minimal instruction residents receive can give them a false sense of mastery.

When factoring residency education into the equation, the overall percentage of time allotted to providing students and young doctors with supervised clinical experience in mental health problems drops to a mere 1 to 3 percent of total teaching time. Educators devote the remaining 97 to 99 percent to diseases and related issues, such as research and statistics. This number persists despite the equal percentages of mental and physical illnesses experienced by patients seeking care.

And it gets worse: practicing physicians often rely on the advice of pharmaceutical sales representatives for how to treat a patient who exhibits signs of mental illness. These representatives have no preparation in mental health or medical care, much less in education. Their sole objective: maximize product sales.

What about training doctors already in practice? As I found in my own experiences, learning the complexities of mental health care demands a huge time expenditure. Even if interested, most physicians cannot take this amount of time for financial and other reasons. Further discouraging, in the only controlled study reporting patient outcomes, the depressed patients demonstrated no improvement when their practicing physicians received training for only one year.[41] Nevertheless, a current one-year training program may hold promise for interested physicians.[42]

Personal Experiences in Medical Education

My personal experiences teaching medical students and residents, I believe, best convey the impact of modern teaching in both its positive and negative dimensions.

A TELLING TEACHING SESSION WITH
RECENT MEDICAL SCHOOL GRADUATES

An experience from one of my classroom seminars with six new interns—an equal mix of male and female first-year residents, all recent graduates from several medical schools—illustrates the impact of medicine's lack of mental health instruction. Not only had their schools foundered in teaching them vital knowledge and skills, but they had also inculcated negative attitudes toward the psychological and social features of care, the "culture of medicine" I mentioned earlier. In the following case I presented to the new residents, see if you can spot the clues to the patient's mental illness that, as you'll soon learn, they missed.

José was a sixty-two-year-old man admitted to the hospital with increasing shortness of breath over the last year and a long history of smoking cigarettes. He had taken his blood pressure medications irregularly and weighed too much. His home doctor had diagnosed diabetes six months earlier, but José rarely took the pills prescribed. He complained that he couldn't concentrate well enough to remember to take them, so he often missed doses. Over the last year, he had lost twelve pounds (without trying) and said it took him more than an hour to get to sleep at night; often he barely slept. His wife told me he didn't enjoy spending time with their grandchildren anymore, and he didn't even want to watch movies, his favorite pastime. The symptoms all began a year ago after he'd been demoted at his job, and they worsened when he learned he didn't qualify for Medicaid.

When I asked the new residents to *identify every health concern that a physician should address*, many ideas arose. Most thought José had emphysema (also called COPD—chronic obstructive pulmonary disease) to explain the shortness of breath. They thought a heart attack or a blood clot in his lungs was unlikely. Some also wondered if he had developed heart failure. Others considered that he might have pneumonia on top of emphysema, which would explain his increased difficulty breathing. A few thought his weight loss could mean that, as a smoker, he had developed lung cancer or, similarly, that his forgetfulness and sleeplessness might mean the cancer had spread to his brain.

After we reviewed the physical examination and all the laboratory and X-ray results, the group agreed he had worsening COPD, poorly controlled diabetes, obesity, and hypertension. They then identified the correct treatment of inhaled aerosols and a short course of prednisone (a steroid). They noted that they would advise José to quit smoking and supply him with nicotine patches to help him with this; finally, they would remind him that he needed to take his medications regularly for his high blood pressure and diabetes.

When I pressed them on whether anything further needed investigation and/or treatment, they drew a blank. I then asked them the specific questions that follow. I include their answers, and the correct answers follow in italics:

- **What about his lack of enjoyment in previously pleasurable activities and his demotion at work a year ago?** They didn't understand the importance of this, and some wondered why I'd asked. *Inability to enjoy life reflects depression, which José developed after his difficulty at work. Both should prompt inquiry about feeling depressed and suicidal.*
- **What about the weight loss and difficulty concentrating and sleeping?** They correctly wondered about the need to look for some other types of cancer. *But such classic symptoms of depression should also prompt inquiry about it.*
- **Why didn't he take his medications?** Most thought he just needed to be told of its importance. *This also is part of being depressed. José lacked the interest and motivation to take his medications.*
- **What about his loss of Medicaid?** None saw the importance of this, and some believed that a social worker should address it, that it simply wasn't a

medical concern. *José couldn't afford the medications, a serious, socially based worry that contributed to his depression.*

When I suggested the importance to good care of recognizing personal difficulties like depression and social issues, such as the inability to afford care, I received a profusion of frustrated and dismissive responses, including the following:

- "That's not my job."
- "I'm prepared in school to treat real diseases, not this touchy-feely stuff."
- "I'm always scared when I hear patients mention these things. I don't know what to do."
- "I didn't go to school to be a psychiatrist."
- "I know these things can be important, but there's not much science behind it. It's more what your mother or grandmother would tell someone to do."
- "I don't like to intrude in others' personal business. It's rude."
- "We were taught to keep our distance from the patient, not to get too close by addressing personal things like this."
- "I see my job as getting all the lab data to make a diagnosis of whatever disease they have; if they don't have one, just tell them nothing is wrong that you can fix. It's as simple as that."

This teaching experience demonstrates two things. First, medical schools teach graduates to recognize and treat organic diseases effectively. Second, these graduates lack the knowledge and skills to recognize and treat mental disorders. Greatly compounding the problem, their attitudes also fall short for treating people with such illnesses as depression. Moreover, their training has not attuned them to social problems such as poverty. This, of course, mirrors their education. But something else lurks inside their education. For example, medical faculty often castigate students and residents if they miss a diagnosis of cancer or heart disease but not for missing a patient's depression or other mental illness. This selective lack of concern reflects a culture of medicine that many experts call the "hidden curriculum."[43]

A Day inside the Teaching Hospital: Evidence of Modern Medical Education's Profound Impact on Patients

I now recount a teaching experience from one day in the hospital where I supervised and taught a team consisting of two third-year medical students, two interns (first-year residents), and one senior resident on one of Michigan State's teaching services in internal medicine—an experience similar to those throughout teaching hospitals in the United States. It offers a series of examples that demonstrate the impact of modern medical training on patients. These cases underline, on the one hand, the positive outcomes for patients with actual diseases and, on the other hand, the ravages imposed on patients with mental disorders.

That day, our teaching team cared for several patients who would not have survived in the past but to whom modern medical care had given a new lease on life. We saw a young woman with Hodgkin's disease (a type of lymph node malignancy)—now cured—who was leaving the hospital that morning to start planning her long-delayed wedding. We also had a young man whose kidney transplant had succeeded. In a couple days, we would discharge him, and he would complete his studies in electrical engineering. A third patient with diabetes had severe pneumonia when admitted to our hospital service. When my group went to see him, he was pacing up and down the hallway; after six days in the hospital, he pleaded with us to let him go home. Given his successful outcome, we discharged him later in the day. These three patients benefited both because of advances in modern medicine and because they had a physical disease, the model of care for which the health care system well prepares its doctors.

But not all our patients fared so well.

GEORGE'S STORY

We had admitted George, a twenty-three-year-old prelaw student, to our hospital service the day before because of an overdose on Xanax, and he had just died in the intensive care unit. Depressed about his prospects for getting into law school, George had taken an overdose of Xanax and never woke up. Twice the preceding week his roommate had taken him to the emergency room because George had complained of feeling depressed; he wouldn't eat, cried frequently, and talked about taking his life. Reading the doctor's emergency room notes from George's first visit, we learned that he had complained of feeling "hopeless" and felt that "life is not worth it." At that time, the doctor gave him the addicting tranquilizer Xanax.

On the second visit, another emergency doctor—still not recognizing either George's depression or his suicidal intent or the perils of Xanax—increased the Xanax dose and reassured George that he "needed to relax; there's more to life than law school anyway." One must wonder, if these emergency room doctors had learned about diagnosing and managing suicidal intent and the proper use of Xanax—a drug absolutely proscribed in a situation like this—would the outcome have changed? *The emergency room doctor should have admitted George to the hospital at the initial visit and referred him to someone skilled in handling acute crises, such as suicidal intent.*

BETSY'S STORY

Then my team saw Betsy, a nineteen-year-old bank clerk. We had admitted her to our care from the emergency room and then transferred her to the intensive care unit. She had overdosed on oxycodone she had found in her mother's medicine cabinet because Betsy wanted to get high with her boyfriend. Betsy's mother had used only three of the ninety pills prescribed for back pain and left the rest in her medicine cabinet. The teen accidentally overdosed; fortunately, her boyfriend had taken only a couple of pills and was able to bring her to the hospital. He said Betsy assumed the pills were safe because they came from a doctor in a prescription bottle—and therefore she took more than the usual one to two pills of the street drugs she sometimes used. The prescribing doctor, an orthopedic physician, was apparently unaware of how to use opioids (they are seldom advised for minor back pain, certainly not in the numbers of pills prescribed). In prescribing opioids, he had inadvertently played a central role in Betsy's now possibly lethal situation. *This illustrates the crucial fact that medicine does not teach its practitioners how to use narcotics or manage pain.*

While seeing our other patients that day, a conversation I had with a new intern on our team, just out of medical school, floored me. I'd asked her why she spent so little time with a depressed sixty-two-year-old man dying of lung cancer. Her answer? "There's nothing I can do. I'd be depressed, too." *But she could do something: prescribe medications for depression and, better still, simply sit with him in a supportive way. Regrettably, she had not learned that she should do this—much less how.*

The next two patients we saw had intertwining physical and mental health disorders. Their mental disorders played a major role in their physical illness, yet their previous physicians overlooked them, focusing entirely on the physical problem.

MOHAMED'S STORY

The emergency room doctors admitted Mohamed, a thirty-four-year-old computer technician, to our hospital service for our teaching team to conduct his care. He complained of spells of chest pain, shortness of breath, feelings of faintness, and profuse sweating. Emergency room doctors at another hospital had admitted him for this same trouble on three earlier occasions in the last month. In addition to much blood work, many electrocardiograms (EKG), and heart- and lung-function monitoring each time, he also received a CAT (computer assisted tomography) scan of his chest to exclude a blood clot in his lungs on each of his first two admissions and, on the third admission, coronary angiograms to exclude a heart attack. All were normal during each of these three- to four-day hospital stays.

When my team first saw him, he was frightened and went on to say about his chest pain and other symptoms, "These just come out of the blue. Am I going to die?" After we reassured him, he gave us the history that made the diagnosis. He said that one moment he felt fine and then, without warning, the symptoms would begin. He reported good health otherwise until about six weeks earlier, when he began to have other difficulties—taking an hour or so to get to sleep and losing interest in his work. When I probed, he became tearful. He said he worried about his family, who lived in an unstable foreign country that had recently undergone great upheaval with fighting and bloodshed and many deaths.

In short, Mohamed had developed a mix of anxiety and depression associated with terrifying panic attacks that repeatedly brought him to the hospital. We initiated treatment for his anxiety and panic attacks and discharged him the same day. We then followed him in our clinic. With medications and the help of a psychologist to treat his panic attacks, he did well. In addition to the needless emotional turmoil he had experienced over that six-week period, I estimate a his four hospitalizations—all avoidable—cost $150,000. *You cannot fault any one doctor in his case; many doctors were involved. The doctors at his first visit to the emergency room should have made the diagnosis of depression with panic attacks and begun effective treatment. The hospitalizations and many tests he endured were not necessary.*

MARIA'S STORY

In a similar example of a mental disorder accompanying a physical illness, we saw sixty-seven-year-old Maria that same day on our hospital teaching service. She had heart failure with shortness of breath and swollen ankles because of a heart attack two years earlier. Her situation had worsened during the preceding year, and doctors had hospitalized her four times in the last two months. Each time she'd improve and feel fine, only to return to the emergency room with the same symptoms a week or two later. The multiple physicians who saw her made no alternate diagnoses and simply advised her to continue her medications and low-salt diet each time.

When we saw her, we soon diagnosed depression. The heart failure prevented her from continuing the activities she enjoyed, such as visiting her grandchildren, going to church, and walking her dog—and her husband would not help her do these activities. He feared she'd die if she exerted herself in any way and wanted her in the hospital. This led her to ignore her diet and stop her medications, saying, "What's the use?" In addition, she indicated having thoughts about dying and said, "That wouldn't be such a bad thing."

We treated her depression with medications, arranged for home assistance with her medications, and outlined in detail an easy walking program. We also met with her husband, reassuring him the low-grade walking we recommended would help her. As her depression cleared, her heart failure remitted because now she had the motivation to stay on her medications and low-salt diet. The following year, she had only one hospitalization. *Again, not one doctor faltered but many. Diseases like heart failure interest the medical system, but mental issues do not, even though clinicians must treat the latter to improve the heart failure itself—as we did with Maria.*

CHAPTER 3

How Patients and Society Suffer

This chapter shows the hardships for patients, their families, and society that ensue from limited access, poor quality, and restricted safety of care for mental health problems. Because these illnesses affect one in four Americans, you or someone you care about may well have experienced the fallout along the lines that follow.

The Prescription-Opioid Crisis

More than 200,000 Americans have died of overdose deaths from *prescribed* opioids since the epidemic began in the 1990s.[1] Only physicians; dentists; and, in some states, psychologists, physician assistants, and nurse practitioners can prescribe highly addicting narcotics. The year 2015 alone saw 18,000 overdose deaths from physician-prescribed narcotics.[2] New regulations have somewhat decreased these national rates, but overdoses on street drugs have increased as a result.[3]

The culprits go by such names as codeine; tramadol; hydrocodone (Norco, Vicodin, Lortab); oxycodone (OxyContin, Roxicodone, Percocet); morphine; fentanyl skin patches; oxymorphone (Opana); hydromorphone (Dilaudid); and narcotic detoxification agents, such as buprenorphine and methadone. Other prescription-only addicting medications are benzodiazepines (Valium, Xanax, Klonopin) and stimulants (Ritalin and Adderall).

You may wonder how the people who have died gained access to all these prescriptions. Although the figure has recently decreased, research from the Centers for Disease Control and Prevention (CDC) reports that in 2013 there were 249,000,000 opioid prescriptions written by doctors, enough for every adult to have his or her own bottle.[4] Another astounding finding from the 2015

National Survey on Drug Use and Health showed that more than one-third of the entire American adult population reported use of a prescription narcotic at some point in their lives.[5]

OPIOID MISUSE

What do people do with nearly 250 million prescriptions? Many misuse them, meaning they take them for *nonprescribed* reasons, such as for recreation ("getting high") or to satisfy an addiction or to give to someone else or even to sell, as opioids are worth a lot on the street.[6] That clinicians—themselves untrained in opioid use—seek to prevent misuse adds another layer of difficulty: They can't determine who is abusing these drugs; it could be the town's coach, banker, or esteemed politician, not just the usual suspects.

BART'S STORY

Bart fooled me. Well dressed and soft-spoken, this forty-four-year-old man came as a new patient to my practice. He wanted to get off the narcotics his previous doctor gave him for now-improved low-back pain—and I believed him. We agreed I'd give him a dose of twenty-one tablets of oxycodone (one tablet three times a day for seven days). This was reduced from what he had been taking—or so he told me. (This occurred before the current prescription-drug-monitoring programs—statewide electronic systems containing all prior addicting medication prescriptions; laws now require that providers check this system before writing new prescriptions or refilling old ones.[7])

    I didn't think any harm could come from such a small dose. I scheduled Bart to see me in a week to reduce his prescription further; we agreed on a goal of stopping the drug over the next several weeks. Well, foolish me. The pharmacy called later that day and said his prescription appeared altered. They asked if I had really prescribed 210 tablets for one week. It turned out that Bart had added a *0* after the number *21* I had written on the prescription form. So no, he didn't come back the following week—he was in jail. I learned that he regularly sold oxycodone and had a long history of going from one doctor to the other for prescriptions.

How bad is this opioid problem? While not everyone who takes narcotics misuses them, each year in America, more than 11 million people do, according to testimony provided to the US Senate Subcommittee on Labor, Health and

Human Services, Education, and Related Agencies.[8] All told, at some point in their lives, 52 million adults have used prescription opioids for nonmedical (nonprescribed) reasons.[9] Especially worrisome, about half of teenagers believe prescription drugs are safe compared to street drugs, preferring them to get high. Still worse, more than half of prescription-drug misusers get them free from a friend or relative.[10] These facts pinpoint where many of the 18,000 deaths from inadvertent overdosing occur.

My personal experiences can put the opioid mishap in perspective. First, during my private practice in the 1970s, I never had to deal with patients demanding narcotics. No one ever requested them, and clinicians only prescribed them for acute problems, such as a fracture, or for patients with chronic problems, such as advanced cancer. But today, things are different. While the United States represents 5 percent of the world's population, Americans consume 75 percent of the world's drugs, as reported by the National Institute of Drug Abuse, the Substance Abuse and Mental Health Services Administration, and others.[11]

In my recent teaching practice, I have worked with many resident doctors from countries outside the United States. The demands of American patients today for narcotics astound them—as do the plentiful quantities American physicians prescribe. For example, one of my clinic residents asked me about a patient's extreme requests: "Dr. Smith, this man wants more oxycodone each month than the total amount of narcotics I prescribed at home during my entire training. I couldn't get them without a special permit. They locked them up. Besides, no one asked for them. What should I do?" The resident's home scenario resembles this country in the 1970s.

ORIGIN OF THE OPIOID EPIDEMIC

In the 1990s, pharmaceutical companies, having developed new narcotics to sell, went all-hands-on-deck to establish a lucrative market of patients with chronic pain. They marketed the drugs to clinicians as safe and effective with expensive, intensive advertising.[12] Drug representatives—who, as you know, had no other training in their use—and all other advertising presented drug-company research as demonstrating the narcotics' safety and effectiveness to doctors. Ubiquitous pharmaceutical representatives frequented physicians' offices and local hospitals. These so-called drug reps offered drug-company information to practitioners about the new narcotics, with OxyContin, the prototype, developed by Purdue Pharma and its physician owners, the Sackler family.[13]

Drug reps have well-honed strategies to gain access to doctors for the purpose of "teaching" them. Through a long tradition in health care, the reps bring gifts to get in the door. On the cheaper end, gifts might range from ballpoint pens and flashlights to a stethoscope or doctor's bag with the drug name on it, to a free lunch with the rep, to free doughnuts and sandwiches for the office staff, who then get the rep on the physician's schedule. At a more expensive level, drug reps threw lavish dinners, where the after-dinner speaker would present an "educational" lecture on long-standing pain and, of course, the new drug's role in managing it. This modus operandi mushroomed into two- to three-day all-expenses-paid vacations to golf resorts called "educational conferences." Speakers paid by the drug company would spend the mornings (afternoons were for the doctors to play golf) discussing the new drug's usefulness in managing prolonged pain. Lucrative monetary payments graced a small group of doctors who gave presentations to other physicians at conferences, where they encouraged the safe use of a new opioid. Indeed, some went "on the circuit" to repeatedly tout drug-company-sponsored research.[14]

Particularly disturbing, the drug reps' gifts, meals, and other freebies granted them an astounding inside track in medical schools. Because of strangely acquiescent medical educators, students and residents in training received reps' drug-company sales pitches *as a seeming part of their education*—typically the only exposure they received in pain management and use of narcotics; indeed, when queried, Massachusetts medical students admitted to feeling unprepared in using narcotics.[15] In teaching hospitals and clinics, pharmaceutical reps regularly bought lunches for groups of faculty and trainees to eat at their daily noon teaching conferences, asking only to have a couple minutes at the end to discuss the new narcotic with the group. In addition to ballpoint pens and mini flashlights, they sometimes left handfuls of already-completed prescription blanks for the narcotic they were marketing, missing only the doctor's signature. The intent was for the doctors to use them with patients later that day.

But more than the pharmaceutical houses created the prescription-narcotic epidemic. During this same period, various pain societies and the influential Joint Commission on the Accreditation of Healthcare Organizations barraged practitioners with information hyping the safe use of opioids and the importance of pain relief for patients; the latter sets accreditation standards for hospitals and other provider organizations.[16] Further compounding the narcotic predicament, the US Congress labeled 2000 to 2010 as the "Decade of Pain Control and Research," and laws regulating prescriptions of addictive medications relaxed.[17] Many doctors, nurses, and others accepted this new view that opioids were safe.

PAIN AS A FIFTH VITAL SIGN

Fostering the opioid crisis, the attitude that clinicians should relieve all pain insidiously supplanted the previous belief about pain as a natural part of healing.[18]

The following illustrates how pervasive this attitude remains even to this day in many hospitals.

The pain societies and governmental agencies promoted the idea that all clinicians and nurses should identify a patient's "fifth vital sign." As you probably know from your own visits, a doctor usually obtains your standard four vital signs: temperature, pulse rate, breathing rate, and blood pressure. Caretakers now added to these four the presence—or absence—of any pain on a one-to-ten scale, where ten is the worst. This means that, for virtually every patient in a medical setting, providers ask if they have pain. If they do, then the new standard required attempts at complete relief.

Good intentions aside, the need to fully eradicate pain greatly magnified the dilemma. For example, regulations require that nurses in US hospitals awaken patients every four hours or so at night to take their five vital signs, and if the slightly awake patient answers "yes" to having any pain, the nurse often requests a prescription for a new narcotic or an increased dose for the one the patient is already taking. My residents on nighttime call duty tell me they hear this request more commonly than any others. Even worse, hospital rules require that, if residents refuse to prescribe the narcotic, they must formally examine the patient—almost always one they have never seen before. So what's easier on a busy night when they already get little sleep: taking thirty to forty minutes to evaluate the patient or thirty seconds on the phone to order a narcotic or increase a dose? Residents pick up the phone and order more drugs.

RECOGNITION THAT OPIOIDS ARE DANGEROUS

But reality struck in the last fifteen years or so, as the adverse impact of prescribed narcotics became increasingly apparent. And clinicians finally recognized that unsound science, blatant misinformation, "expert" opinion, and uncontrolled observations from the flawed research that characterizes drug-company advertising.[19]

Extensive, rigorous, and independent research, reviewed and summarized by the National Academies of Sciences, Engineering, and Medicine and the CDC, demonstrated *no proven benefit from opioid use in chronic noncancer pain*, the most common reason for prescribing them.[20] Based on an extensive database of reliable research, the CDC and others recently advised that clinicians *initiate* narcotic use only for acute pain—and for no more than three to seven days.[21]

Not only does rigorous research show little or no value from opioids for chronic pain, but it also demonstrates that, in addition to the tragedy of overdose deaths and the terrible complications from addiction and dependence, narcotics cause much distress because of their powerful side effects: reduced sexual function, severe constipation, falls and fractures, lack of motivation, and mental confusion.[22]

Ironically, narcotics sometimes make pain *worse*. First, they induce depression in patients taking these drugs, and that in itself worsens the pain.[23] Second, in a condition known as opioid hyperalgesia, continuously prescribed opioids reset the brain's pain-related chemical receptors, so the body paradoxically becomes more sensitive to pain.[24] My experience in my teaching team's clinic at Michigan State corroborates this.[25] Patients' pain often improves when we treat the depression and reduce or stop the narcotic!

Unfortunately, the guidelines from the CDC that physicians curtail initiating narcotics triggered a new dilemma. Many clinicians regrettably misinterpreted this recommendation to mean that those patients already addicted and dependent on opioids should reduce their drug dosage and/or discontinue them altogether. When doctors terminated or markedly reduced these drugs, patients endured bodily and psychological withdrawal of significant, sometimes lethal proportions.[26]

Experts, including those who wrote the initial CDC guidelines, have reemphasized that, in most cases of those already addicted to or otherwise dependent on prescribed opioids, clinicians should reduce the dose only as tolerated to reach a safe level. However, some patients cannot handle a decreased dose. While taking other measures to treat their addiction, they must stay at higher doses. At the same time, doctors should not abandon these patients, as some have done.[27]

This poses a terribly difficult situation for practitioners: They now face thousands of patients dependent on narcotics who want to acquire them for legitimate use and equal numbers of those who will misuse them—nearly all of whom demand refills vociferously.[28] The opioid mess itself is compounded by doctors' lack of preparation to manage those dependent on opioids; in addition, educators have not taught students and residents to handle demanding, angry patients, and doctors often write prescriptions as an alternative to facing such conflict.

A COMPLEX, NEW ISSUE EMERGES: CHRONIC PAIN

Yet I believe that the more fundamental defect is that *schools have not prepared physicians to manage chronic pain*, the reason for most long-term narcotic prescriptions. Chronic pain may be located almost anywhere in the body (often low back, neck, muscular, pelvic, abdominal, or head) and is defined as lasting six months or more.[29] Although often lacking a clear disease explanation in such conditions as fibromyalgia or irritable bowel syndrome, the pain also may stem from chronic physical disorders: for example, cancer, diabetic nerve damage, sickle cell anemia, or arthritis. But there is more to it.

Chronic pain often results in significant disability, making patients unable to function normally and enjoy life. They lose a great deal in their lives: for example, the ability to work, play golf, go to church, attend school, have sex, have healthy relationships, and simply relax. With such incapacity, the disorder typically leads to a mental illness. Why the onset of psychological problems? Understandably, such anguish and adversity make many people depressed or anxious and inclined to seek any relief possible, including narcotics, alcohol, or other dangerous substances.

I have found chronic pain the most difficult of all medical and mental health disorders to treat—and to teach students and doctors to manage. It requires, in addition to medical skills in diagnosis, skills in handling patients' psychological and social problems that most physicians lack for treatment. For example, they do not know how to use depression and anxiety medications and often think it proper to initiate opioids—and they do not know how to manage someone already taking them.

The Suicide Crisis

In 2018, the number of suicides reached 48,000, up from nearly 43,000 in 2014.[30] Although, suicide occurs more commonly in the older community, the recent increases disproportionately involve young people, as well as those with low levels of education and those with mental disorders.[31] Sadly, clinicians have little if any training in recognizing and managing the crises these patients represent.

Thankfully, recent interventions from the National Suicide Prevention Lifeline show promise; since July 2022, a new hotline (call 988) is available across the United States.[32] Not including the United States, an international study demonstrated that such national prevention programs make a significant dent in the horrific number of suicides taking place in men aged twenty-five to sixty-four and in women aged forty-five to greater than sixty-five years old.[33]

But practitioners can prevent far more suicides than they have in the past. Again, the frontline care individuals receive comes to the fore. Nearly half—45 percent—of patients who commit suicide visit their medical doctor in the thirty days before their deaths, and as many as 75 percent consult them during the preceding year.[34] Within the especially vulnerable population of troubled alcohol users, almost 40 percent who died of suicide consulted their physician in the two weeks preceding death, according to a large national study in Sweden.[35]

I know you will find it difficult to believe, but educational programs struggle in preparing doctors to recognize (diagnose) the suicidal patient, much less teach its management. Educators have viewed suicide as a low priority for medicine.[36]

Understandably defensive medical school deans and residency program directors will argue vigorously that they do address suicide and opioids. Once you pin them down, however, you'll discover they present the topics in just a couple lectures here and there. They proffer no intensive, supervised curriculum involving actual distressed patients that allow students and residents to learn how to address these death traps for so many Americans.[37] Their priorities resound.

The Crisis in Depression and Anxiety Disorders

Lamentably, adversity extends considerably beyond death resulting from overdose or suicide. Americans experience far more prevalent nonlethal consequences from psychological illnesses—depression and anxiety disorders foremost—as reported by the American Psychiatric Association's *Diagnostic and Statistical Manual of Mental Disorders* (5th edition).[38]

Physicians usually ignore patients' symptoms of these diagnoses: for example, low mood, fatigue, insomnia, worry, agitation, despair, and hopelessness. They also overlook the conditions that should prompt them to inquire about these symptoms, such as divorce and strained relationships, impaired school and job performance, lower socioeconomic status, homelessness, criminality, refractory pain or other debilitating medical condition, and alcohol and drug use. These oversights preclude implementing the highly effective treatments now available. Yet the right treatment can turn a life around, as I show in a couple case reports.

But first, I'm embarrassed to present an example of this national impasse of poor recognition from my own clinics. Unique in American primary care, our teaching team at Michigan State set up a mental health clinic within the internal medicine clinic where Michigan State clinicians see all patients. This exposed a huge gap in care, paralleling a well-known shortfall across the country. As part of providing mental health consultation to our medical colleagues, my team evaluated the patients they referred to our clinic. *Shocking* understates what we observed. The patients had received care in our medical clinics for most, if not all, of their primary and other health care for nearly six years on average. What about the severity of their mental illnesses? They averaged 2.3 major psychiatric diagnoses per person, mostly related to depression, anxiety, and chronic pain.[39] Yet only 12 percent had ever seen a psychiatrist, and fewer than 30 percent had seen any mental health specialist at all—even once—during the entire course of six years under the clinic's care.

I can't relate these recent histories due to confidentiality, but two similar examples from my earlier experiences illustrate the types of mental illnesses overlooked in primary care and other medical settings—and how recognizing and treating the illness can transform a troubled life into a happy, successful one.

BEN'S STORY

Ben was a seventy-two-year-old man referred to me for a physical examination that regulations required before he could be admitted to an institution for Alzheimer's disease—at least that's the illness the neurologist and primary care physician had given as the explanation for the profound changes he exhibited. Ben couldn't recall his own phone number, the president's name, or the date; on this cold winter day, he answered, "May."

In conversation with his daughter, I learned that he'd also had several crying spells and couldn't sleep at night. Speaking with her further, I found that Ben's symptoms had begun shortly after the death of his wife—less than two years earlier—and progressively worsened. His daughter wondered if this had anything to do with his faltering memory. So did I. In speaking with Ben for nearly an hour, he eventually said that he felt "kind of down" and missed his wife so much that "nothing's worth it anymore." Later he mentioned thinking about taking his life with some Xanax his wife had received before she died. I also learned that he'd been perfectly well before her death and that he knew the month was, in fact, January.

After ruling out several other conditions, I made a diagnosis of pseudodementia, which means depression causing symptoms of apparent dementia. My team treated his depression over a long period of time in the hospital and then with intensive counseling by a psychologist as an outpatient. Ever so slowly, he returned to normal over the next twelve months. In the end, Ben was not placed in an institution, and the following year, he even returned to playing some golf. No one had thought to investigate depression. Even though he suffered greatly, the outcome for Ben could have been far worse.

JANINE'S STORY

Janine was a thirty-nine-year-old mid-level executive who had worked mostly in the field providing hands-on supervision of her internet technology group. Her success led to an offer for a position where she would instruct others on how to run similar groups. Janine regarded the role somewhat reluctantly; she didn't like to speak in front of groups, and shyness and nervousness had always troubled her. However, she accepted the job in a major advancement.

Unfortunately, Janine's apprehension about the job proved correct. Her anxiety continued to grow, not just when speaking to groups, and the company doctor gave her Valium, but this just made her sleepy. She also couldn't concentrate, and her presentations and other work consequently faltered. Even with the Valium, she noted ongoing anxiety and trouble sleeping and waking, and she found herself worrying about the next day. When Janine first came to my clinic, she tearfully admitted, "I just can't do this any longer. I'm quitting and going back to my old job."

With medications and counseling by a psychologist, we successfully treated Janine's anxiety disorder. I also gave her a nonaddicting medication (propranolol) to lessen her reaction to the anxiety, and over about eight weeks, she slowly stopped the Valium. Some time has passed, so I know the happy ending. Janine improved not only with treatment but also with experience and ongoing counseling by her psychologist. She became more confident in speaking and presenting, eventually getting off the medications. No, she didn't rise to her company's presidency, but she enjoyed her work—a real-life remodeling that her doctors almost scuttled.

━━◆━━

In short, health care must address the human condition—suffering—whether that derives from a bodily or psychological disorder. In both Ben's and Janine's cases, recognizing and treating the mental disorder had a profound influence on the patient's entire life. Such impact is no less important than recognizing and correctly treating someone's pneumonia, appendicitis, hip fracture, or heart attack.

The Dire Effects of COVID-19 on Mental Health

Patients have suffered an extraordinary degree of angst because of COVID-19. In addition to the deadly virus itself, Americans have also experienced vastly increased diagnoses of depression, anxiety, and substance abuse. And almost all of these have been managed by inexperienced clinicians.

Research tells a woeful tale. In March 2020—still early in the pandemic—when Kaiser Family Foundation investigators asked a large group of adults "if their mental health had been negatively impacted due to worry and stress by the virus," 32 percent answered yes. By August of the same year, the rate rose to 53 percent.[40] This means that more than half the US population described being in severe distress. And during this same time period, the CDC reported that 13 percent either began or increased their use of alcohol. Even more frightening, the CDC found that 10.7 percent of the population responded that they had "seriously considered suicide" in the previous thirty days. The numbers for this response were especially high in African Americans (15.1 percent), Hispanics (18.6 percent), essential workers (21.7 percent), young people (25.5 percent), and unpaid caregivers (30.7 percent).[41]

Children and adolescents also did not escape the coronavirus's ravages, according to a recent report.[42] Research that synthesized twenty-nine studies (called a meta-analysis) evaluated more than 80,000 youths from East Asia, North America, Europe, Central America, South America, and the Middle East during the pandemic's first year. One in four experienced depression, and one in five, anxiety, approximately doubling prepandemic rates.

Many adults also experienced a dramatic increase in developing new psychological illnesses. In 2019, before the pandemic, 11 percent of adults had symptoms suggesting a major anxiety or depressive disorder. During the pandemic in 2020, the rate increased to 36–41 percent, depending on the month, according to CDC research—a tripling or quadrupling. This means that the virus-induced stress caused more than 80 million Americans to develop a *new* mental disorder—a fact almost beyond comprehension.[43] COVID-19 also worsened an even greater percentage of patients with an *existing psychiatric illness*. And the toll I've described does not even include the devastation, especially depression, experienced by those infected by the virus, with its attendant isolation, fear, and often limited help.[44]

The Crisis in Chronic Physical Diseases

Surprisingly, actual disease care—medicine's forte—also stands on shaky ground. Chronic physical diseases, such as heart disease, diabetes, and cancer, have accompanying psychological and social factors that doctors must address to effectively care for the disease. But medicine does not do this, leading to the crisis of substandard physical-disease care.

The problem arose when the US patient population began to morph from acute to chronic diseases in the mid-twentieth century because the latter required attention to psychosocial factors.[45] Although acute illnesses also had coexisting mental and psychosocial elements, ignoring them made little difference, because with acute illness, it either quickly resolved, or the patient died. Not so with protracted physical diseases—now health care's most common diagnosis—because successful treatment required integration of psychological and social issues into care, as you will soon see.[46]

First, though, to understand the failure in chronic diseases, it helps to appreciate what happened to Americans' health care needs over the last century. Note in table 3.1 the predominance of such acute diseases as pneumonia, tuberculosis,

Table 3.1.   Leading Causes of Death in the United States in 1900 and 1997, in Order of Frequency

1900	1997
Tuberculosis	Heart disease
Pneumonia	Cancer
Diarrhea	Stroke
Heart disease	Chronic lung disease
Liver disease	Unintentional injuries
Injuries	Pneumonia/influenza
Stroke	Diabetes
Cancer	Suicide
Bronchitis	Chronic kidney disease
Diphtheria	Chronic liver disease

and diarrheal disorders, all infectious diseases, as the main causes of death in 1900; by 1997, the chronic disease killers so familiar today (heart disease, cancer, stroke, and lung disease) have almost entirely replaced them.[47] Except for suicide, unintentional injuries, and pneumonia/influenza, all conditions listed in 1997 are chronic diseases. Indeed, according to the CDC, by 2022, six of the top seven causes of death stemmed from chronic diseases. Heart disease and cancer accounted for nearly half of them, but stroke, diabetes, Alzheimer's disease, and lung disease also rated high.[48] CDC research showed that six of ten adults have at least one chronic disease, while four of ten experience two or more.[49]

Three chronic disease scenarios represent the need for fully integrating psychosocial factors into medicine: (1) chronic disorders with an accompanying mental illness, (2) chronic illnesses caused by psychosocial and emotional features unrelated to a mental illness, and (3) patients' psychosocially based nonadherence to treatment recommendations in chronic diseases.

CHRONIC DISORDERS WITH AN ACCOMPANYING MENTAL ILLNESS

Long-standing physical disorders frequently have co-occurring mental disorders. According to research from the Robert Wood Johnson Foundation, some 17 percent of adults in the United States (30 million) suffer from this condition.[50] When a psychological illness exists alongside a chronic disease, a patient commonly endures more severe disability, work absences, and reductions in quality of life—and greater costs.[51] And death rates are six times higher than in people with neither disorder and two times higher than in those with just one or the other disorder.[52] In patients with a chronic disorder and a mental illness, disease care itself falters if clinicians do not identify and treat the associated psychiatric disorder.

You may wonder why mental illnesses and medical diseases co-occur. Either one may lead to the other.[53] First, a mental disorder can cause a physical disease.[54] For example, depression can push a patient to overeat and smoke cigarettes, and he or she may become obese and develop diabetes and heart disease. Depression is closely associated with the subsequent development of cardiovascular diseases, according to recent reports.[55] More generally, a history of any psychopathology correlates strongly with the premature onset of age-related diseases, such as stroke and heart disease.[56]

Second, the process can work in reverse: Physical illness can trigger a mental disorder.[57] Understandably, if a person can no longer go to church or work or visit with relatives because of incapacity from diabetes, persistent pain, or cancer, then that person can become depressed or anxious or start to abuse addicting substances.[58] Unfortunately, research from the United Kingdom demonstrates that, when patients with common cancers develop depression, survival falls significantly.[59]

Which comes first, however, makes no difference for treatment. Experts tell us that, whether the mental illness precedes or follows the physical disease, treatment succeeds to a much greater extent when the clinician treats the depression or other mental disorder while simultaneously attending to the bodily disease itself.[60] Here's an example of what happens when an unrecognized mental disorder coexists with a chronic disease—and how diagnosing and treating the mental illness can salvage a patient's life.

CLARENCE'S STORY

My teaching team of Michigan State residents and students admitted sixty-year-old Clarence to our hospital service with "brittle" diabetes, which is a type difficult to control. Due to irregularities in how he took his insulin and his difficulty in following other instructions for care, such as diet and blood testing, his blood sugars varied widely from high to low at different times. Clarence had been admitted to another hospital three times in the preceding six weeks due to unconsciousness from low blood sugars, a condition known as hypoglycemia. Low blood sugars can cause death or, if the patient survives, severe brain damage. His out-of-control diabetes put him at considerable risk, and my team realized he would need close attention.

My resident spotted the cause immediately. She asked Clarence about his mood, and he replied, "Low as a snake since my wife died last year." In brief, we treated his severe depression, as well as his diabetes, and followed up with him in our clinic after discharging him from the hospital. Over the next six months, Clarence's mood slowly brightened, but something else happened. His diabetes also came under good control, with no more episodes of low blood sugars or admissions to the hospital. Why the turnabout in his diabetes, his chronic disease? Severe depression overrode the motivation and concentration Clarence needed to attend to his health, which led him to not take his insulin regularly or follow his diet.

In a supreme irony, modern care eschews mental disorders to focus on physical diseases, but this unidimensional interest impairs disease care itself in the 30 million people who have both disorders. Why? *It is only when clinicians treat a coexisting mental disorder that the chronic disease itself maximally improves.*[61] Here's the issue: Modern clinicians rarely employ evidence-based treatments for psychiatric illnesses accompanying chronic diseases.[62] This leads them oftentimes to label these patients "complex" to explain their poor outcomes.[63]

CHRONIC DISEASES CAUSED BY PSYCHOSOCIAL FEATURES UNRELATED TO A MENTAL ILLNESS

Nearly all chronic physical disorders are caused by psychosocial lifestyle issues unrelated to a mental disorder. These include overeating, not exercising, smoking cigarettes, and using alcohol or street drugs. They cause a wide range of diseases, including heart attacks, strokes, cancer, obesity, diabetes, liver disease, drug addiction, and emphysema.[64] Addressing these psychosocial factors is crucial for effective treatment of these diseases, but that can be particularly difficult because this requires that clinicians convince patients to revamp their lifestyles in ways they probably don't want to do—eat less, exercise, quit smoking, and stop using addictive substances.

Here's a fact about lifestyle issues many don't know: *One can prevent most chronic diseases by not adopting or by discontinuing the adverse lifestyle that produces them.* The Partnership to Fight Chronic Disease estimates that, if patients established healthy lifestyles, 80 percent of all cardiovascular diseases (such as heart disease and strokes), 80 percent of all diabetes, and 40 percent of all cancers could be prevented.[65] As physician-author Robert Pearl laments, medicine waits until such avoidable diseases take root and only then treats them, at inordinately greater cost to individuals and to the society that pays for health care.[66] A recent report indicates that, from the $4.3 trillion health care expenditures in 2022, only 4.4 percent went to public health and prevention.[67]

CHRONIC DISORDERS AND NONADHERENCE TO TREATMENT

Another psychosocial issue that is unrelated to lifestyle or mental illness plays a key role in determining outcomes of diseases, namely a patient's adherence to treatment recommendations. Everyone knows that treatment requires that patients comply if it is to be effective. Now, think about how much difficulty you or your family may have had in taking a prescription—without missing doses—for just a week or so. Then, consider that the person with a prolonged disease must frequently keep track of and take ten or more medications over years, even decades. Not surprisingly, this same research indicates that 30 to 50 percent of patients do not take their medications as prescribed. That poses a huge concern.[68]

Providers fall flat in diagnosing nonadherence and thereby don't address or correct it. Physicians and families often blame patients for not following instructions, but patients do not take their medications for a host of understandable reasons: expense, lack of understanding or attentiveness, or a belief it doesn't work and/or results in harm.[69] Rather than blaming patients, physicians must engage patients at the personal and social levels and try to understand their motivations, emotions, and beliefs that lead them to stray from following recommendations.[70]

While some doctors today do advise patients on matters of lifestyle change and medication adherence, getting patients to change depends on doing far more than offering simple admonitions, such as "You need to get more exercise," "You should stop smoking," or "Be sure to take your medicines like I told you to." Rather, it takes a doctor with patient-centered skills, one who knows how to inform and motivate patients. This ability requires good communication with a patient over a period of time and must be based on a strong relationship.

Unfortunately, some assume that patient-centeredness simply means extending common courtesies to patients in a respectful way, but in fact, being nice is just the beginning. Clinicians need to learn intricate, often counterintuitive patient-centered skills: for example, allowing the patient some control of the interaction while maintaining effective and efficient care; motivating patients to do something they prefer not to do; negotiating rather than prescribing alternative lifestyle habits; and accepting a decision by the patient not to follow advice. Teaching these skills is labor and time-intensive, as I know through my years of doing this at the University of Rochester and Michigan State University. It takes time and repeated practice under expert supervision.

The Crisis in Cost

According to health care economics expert Stephen Melek and colleagues, patients with coexisting mental and chronic physical disorders cost up to three times more to treat than chronic-disease patients with no associated mental illness; this is especially true of those with long-standing and severe illnesses.[71] While they represent only about 5 percent of the patient population, patients with co-occurring mental and physical disorders account for about one-half of all spending on present health care—a good place to start if the United States hopes to save health care dollars.[72]

Surprisingly, about 80 percent of this extra expense derives from increased expenditures caused by the disease, such as the patient having to be readmitted repeatedly to the hospital or the patient's failure to comply with treatment instructions, particularly medication adherence and follow-up visits to the physician.[73] Melek and Norris compared nondepressed physical-disease patients to those with an associated depression diagnosis, and the latter cost more than $6,000 per year additionally.[74]

Now do the math. Recalling that 30 million people with chronic diseases have an associated mental illness in any twelve-month period, this comes to nearly $200 billion a year in excess medical costs. Sadly, the authors report that only 12.7 percent of patients received even minimally adequate treatment for depression accompanying medical diseases.[75]

Although the nation suffers financially from huge health care expenses, research done by Melek and his colleagues creates a ray of hope. In careful cost analyses, they found that the United States could *save* between $26 billion and $48 billion *yearly* by integrating care in patients with chronic diseases and associated mental illnesses.[76] These savings could support the entire National Institutes of Health (NIH), whose budget for 2017 was about $32.6 billion.[77]

I said earlier that the United States could reduce its massive annual health care budget by as much as trillions of dollars, but what I've presented so far does not come close to that, even if I include correcting nonadherence to medications, whose estimated savings would be approximately $100 billion per year.[78] Stay tuned. Recall that chronic disease patients have lifestyle factors that lead to far, far greater expenses. Chronic diseases are today's most common problem, causing 70 percent of all deaths and accounting for 81 percent of all hospital admissions. Not surprisingly, they also account for the greatest health care expenses. In a system spending $3.8 trillion in 2019 and $4.5 trillion in 2022, chronic diseases lead to 75 percent of all spending and 99 percent of all Medicare spending.[79]

Taxpayers can hit the jackpot here. I mentioned earlier that the public and medicine working together could *prevent* 40–80 percent of chronic diseases by changing the patient's psychosocially based lifestyle habits.[80] By preventing uptake of adverse health habits or helping patients to successfully discontinue such habits if already adopted, the United States can save *trillions* of dollars. Given that recent yearly health care expenditures have ranged from $3.8 trillion to $4.5 trillion, savings could be *$1–2 trillion every year* simply from effectively implementing the strategy. That's *$10–20 trillion in ten years*. But this will require, in addition to much more vigorous public health efforts, medical schools to train physicians in preventive practices based on such patient-centered efforts as I note in this chapter.[81]

Part II

THE MIND-BODY SPLIT

CHAPTER 4

The Origins of the Mind-Body Split

There is a fascinating story of why medicine discarded its patients' psychological and social dimensions in favor of an isolated focus on their physical diseases. Known as the mind-body split, three historical factors led medicine to jettison mental health and other mind-related issues. This chapter addresses the split's origin in anatomy in the sixteenth century at the start of the Scientific Revolution; the next chapter describes how it became firmly established by such philosophers as Descartes a century later—and how, in the nineteenth century, as clinicians began to associate patients' symptoms with what autopsies revealed about diseases, the split became intrinsic to actual patient care.

The most basic of the medical sciences of the sixteenth century—human anatomy—launched the Scientific Revolution, and this is where the mind-body split began. But it was the then all-powerful Catholic Church's view of the mind that actually caused it. The church believed the mind, spirit, and soul were contained in the head, and the head was the church's domain, not medicine's. The result was that, although the church allowed human dissections for teaching physicians, it required that anatomists restrict their dissections to the parts of the body below the head—from the neck down. This led medical science to ignore the brain and mind. Until this time, from the beginning of scientific medicine with Hippocrates in the fifth century BC through the fifteenth century AD, medical science had integrated the mind and body as one. The inception of a mind-body duality in the sixteenth century initiated a radical revolution that would gradually spread throughout the basic sciences and much later permeate clinical practice. Appendix A summarizes the evolution of the mind-body duality I describe over this and the following chapter.

Hippocrates and the Dawn of Scientific Medicine

Scientific medicine dawns with the Greeks in the fifth century BC and is the starting point at which we can evaluate attention to mind and mental illnesses in medical care. The eminent medical historians Fielding Garrison and Roy Porter have said that Hippocrates crystallized the loose knowledge of prior schools to create the first systematic science of medicine in the West.[1] Hippocrates was born on the island of Kos and lived from 460 to 377 BC in the classic period, the age of Pericles.[2] Today we know Hippocrates's works mainly through the sixty to seventy books of his corpus, written mostly, if not entirely, by his many followers and their students.[3]

Hippocrates dissociated the profession from religion and rejected the superstition that diseases were punishments from the various Greek gods.[4] He argued that the same scientific laws that described the cosmos also governed humankind. Hippocrates believed that health care should be rational and based on an empirical understanding of the body in its natural environment.[5] His appeal to reason reflected Greek attitudes generally.[6]

Hippocratic medicine united the mind and body in patient care, presenting a holistic perspective.[7] Greek clinicians saw no reason to separate patients' mental and physical elements, viewing them as a single unit. Practitioners incorporated mental disorders into medicine, recognizing melancholia and mania, for example, as part of everyday health care. Hippocrates propounded trust between doctor and patient and believed that a diagnosis required looking beyond a given disease to include the patient's way of life, habits, work, and even diet.[8]

Textboxes 4.1 and 4.2 offer some of Hippocrates's clinical descriptions of patients and various disorders he identified.[9] I find it amazing that his work remains applicable more than two millennia later. Justifiably, many called Hippocrates the "father of medicine," and given his contributions, many go so far as to label him the "greatest of all physicians."[10] I certainly agree, mainly because of his conceptualization of a united mind and body, the message of this book.

Textbox 4.1. Clinical Descriptions of Patients by Hippocrates

1. **Hippocratic fingers:** clubbed appearance of fingertips and fingernails that suggest such lung problems as tuberculosis and cancer
2. **Hippocratic facies:** the facial appearance of a dying person
3. **Hippocratic smile:** not really a smile; rather, the grimace of patients with tetanus
4. **Succussion splash:** the splashing sound made when a clinician vigorously shakes the chest (or abdomen) of a patient who has a large collection of fluid in the lungs (or stomach)

Textbox 4.2. Disorders Identified by Hippocrates

1. **Phthisis:** tuberculosis; the name reflects the progressive wasting (i.e., consumption) of a person with tuberculosis
2. **Melancholia:** depression
3. **Mania:** bipolar disorder
4. **Puerperal sepsis:** maternal infection following childbirth
5. **Epilepsy**
6. **Epidemic parotitis:** mumps
7. **Malaria**
8. **Anthrax**

Hippocrates also insisted on moral, humane conduct by the physician.[11] Textbox 4.3 presents the most famous portion of his corpus, the Hippocratic Oath. It carved out a lofty role for the selfless physician.[12] Today students still take this pledge upon graduation, albeit in modernized forms.[13] Indeed, an enduring legacy.

Textbox 4.3. The Hippocratic Oath

I swear by Apollo Physician and Asclepius and Hygieia and Panaceia and all the gods and goddesses, making them my witnesses, that I will fulfill according to my ability and judgment this oath and this covenant:

To hold him who has taught me this art as equal to my parents and to live my life in partnership with him, and if he is in need of money to give him a share of mine, and to regard his offspring as equal to my brothers in male lineage and to teach them this art—if they desire to learn it—without fee and covenant; to give a share of precepts and oral instruction and all the other learning to my sons and to the sons of him who has instructed me and to pupils who have signed the covenant and have taken an oath according to the medical law, but to no one else.

I will apply dietetic measures for the benefit of the sick according to my ability and judgment; I will keep them from harm and injustice.

I will neither give a deadly drug to anybody if asked for it, nor will I make a suggestion to this effect. Similarly, I will not give to a woman an abortive remedy. In purity and holiness, I will guard my life and my art.

I will not use the knife, not even on sufferers from stone, but will withdraw in favor of such men as are engaged in this work.

Whatever houses I may visit, I will come for the benefit of the sick, remaining free of all intentional injustice, of all mischief, and in particular of sexual relations with both female and male persons, be they free or slaves.

What I may see or hear in the course of the treatment or even outside of the treatment in regard to the life of men, which on no account one must spread abroad, I will keep to myself holding such things shameful to be spoken about.

If I fulfill this oath and do not violate it, may it be granted to me to enjoy life and art, being honored with fame among all men for all my time to come; if I transgress it and swear falsely, may the opposite of all this be my lot.

Hippocrates's rational approach mirrored that of his society. The ancient Greeks were the first civilized people with sufficient leisure time to cultivate the intellect, and they perceived the mind as central to society's workings intellectually, politically, culturally, and artistically.[14] The Greeks had emerged newly sensitive and introspective from the previous warlike attitudes of their battling city-states.[15] Their insights into the mind and behavior impressively survive to form the basis of some of our greatest plays, such as Sophocles's *Oedipus Rex* and *Antigone*; exquisite works of art, pottery, metalwork, and sculpture, such as the *Venus de Milo*; and remarkable architecture—extraordinary theaters, temples, and coliseums, such as Athens's Parthenon. Greek ideas would influence many in the arts and sciences down through the ages.[16]

Nevertheless, in spite of the achievements of Hippocrates's new medicine, there were many weaknesses.[17] Greek doctors had little knowledge of the body's inner workings. Their organizing concept of health and illness was that imbalances of the body's four fluid humors (phlegm, blood, yellow bile, and black bile) represented diseases and led to patients' symptoms.[18] As you will see, this concept of disease would guide clinical medical practices until the nineteenth century AD, including its practice of bloodletting as a treatment for restoring balance to disrupted humors.[19] While Greek physicians understood surface anatomy and did experimental work dissecting animals, society forbade human dissection.[20]

A Long Dry Spell for Medicine

It took almost seven hundred years for medicine to take its next leap forward. Another great Greek physician emerged in the second century AD: Galen of Pergamon. Galen, who lived from 131 to 201 AD, was a Christian and combined his own concept of spirit with Hippocrates's idea of four humors and the ancient Greek idea of illness as punishment. But Galen viewed the symptoms as punishment coming from the Christian God rather than the Greek gods of Hippocratic times.[21] He also replaced Hippocrates's openness and spirit of inquiry with rigid church-based doctrine.[22] Nevertheless, like Hippocrates, Galen regarded the mind and body as a single entity.[23] He ascribed diagnoses of melancholia and mania to alterations in the four humors and believed body and mind affected one another—the two inextricably linked. The mind remained central to him and to those practitioners who came after him.[24]

Galen's work was especially important because it would guide medicine for more than a millennium. He made massive contributions to understanding the body's internal mechanisms. Galen set Hippocratic principles within a wider anatomical and physiological framework by conducting extensive animal dissections and research.[25] One of the first to conduct scientific experiments, Galen made valuable contributions to understanding the circulation of blood to and from the heart.[26] A fine clinician, he also believed the patient's trust was essential and that doctors could win it by a careful bedside manner and clearly explaining the person's illness.[27] Galen authored 350 titles, more than all other Greek writers combined.[28]

Galenic medicine fit nicely with the governing Christian tradition, which viewed the benefits of medical care as the bounty of God—and disease as God inflicting punishment for some social or spiritual transgression. With his sectarian slant, Galen became the predominant figure in Western medical thinking, while Hippocrates's secular, reasoned method lost favor.

To understand the mind-body dichotomy that would come many years later requires an appreciation of the Catholic Church's extraordinary power throughout the thousand-year period between Galen and the Scientific Revolution. In the fifth century AD, Emperor Constantine established Christianity as the empire's only religion. Science and health care progressively fell under complete domination by the church. As a result, the scientific vantage point flagged.[29] Thus few medical advances occurred in Europe during the thousand years following Galen—an era often called the dark ages of medicine.[30] Indeed, Galen's writings governed medical practices for more than a millennium after his death.[31] With the sixteenth-century Scientific Revolution, however, medical thinking changed radically.

The Sixteenth-Century Scientific Revolution

To get a good grasp of how medicine lost its connection to the mind, one must look at the centerpiece of science in the sixteenth century: the study of human anatomy and the attendant need for dissecting the human body. Church policies on human dissections played a key role in the initial mind-body separation. Although scientists had always viewed anatomy as the most basic science, human dissections rarely took place before the Scientific Revolution.[32] Except for a brief period during the third century BC, when anatomists frequently performed them, the practice waned as Christianity became widespread. The Catholic Church judged human dissections immoral and prohibited them, and they eventually disappeared altogether.[33] Instead, scientists relied on dissecting the bodies of cows, pigs, goats, and sheep, believing—erroneously—that they represented human anatomy,

However, pressured by a burgeoning and increasingly powerful scientific community, Pope Clement in Rome finally relented and approved human dissections for teaching anatomy to physicians in 1537 AD.[34] But he imposed the stumbling block that initiated the mind-body split. As mentioned earlier, Catholic authorities regarded the human body's head as sacrosanct.[35] Consequently, before a dissection could proceed, scientists had to decapitate the corpse and literally turn the head over to the church.[36] Scientists thus could not tamper with the soul and mind.[37]

With the head removed, scientists could not evaluate the brain. But even more importantly, the symbolic ramifications exceeded this physical restriction. Scientists could not address the workings of the mind or any other features concerning it, such as emotions and mental health; they belonged with the church. By default, scientists restricted their focus to human beings' nonmental features, the part of the body below the head. This set a precedent for anatomists and, in turn, other human sciences that would soon flourish, such as physiology and chemistry.

THE SCIENTIFIC REVOLUTION BEGINS: ANDREAS VESALIUS

Flemish physician Andreas Vesalius (1514–1564) awakened the scientific world and launched modern medical science with his *De humani corporis fabrica* (*On the Fabric of the Human Body*), known as the *Fabrica*, published in 1543.[38] Born into a celebrated family of doctors, Vesalius carefully and painstakingly conducted extensive human dissections—even going so far as robbing the graves of newly buried dead.[39]

I'll describe Vesalius's remarkable successes shortly, but it's first interesting to understand why he succeeded where previous sixteenth-century anatomists had not: he performed the dissections himself.[40] In contrast, earlier anatomists did not execute their own human dissections, as figure 4.1 depicts. Rather, they lectured to their students from a distant podium using Galen's texts, while a second person, usually a barber surgeon, conducted the actual dissection of the body.[41] A third person pointed out the anatomical structures the lecturing anatomist described. This procedure simply replicated Galen's one-thousand-year-old teachings. To quote Vesalius from the *Fabrica* on this earlier practice,

> The deplorable method of instruction which is used today demands that one person—generally a surgeon or barber—should carry out the dissection of the human body, while the lecturer reads a description of the different parts of the anatomy derived from books. . . . Those who are actually performing the dissection are so ignorant that they are in fact not in a position to demonstrate to the students the parts they are preparing, or to explain them, and as the professor never touches the corpse and as the dissector does not know the Latin names and therefore cannot follow the lecture in sequence, each goes his own way. . . . In the confusion the student learns less than a butcher could teach the professor.[42]

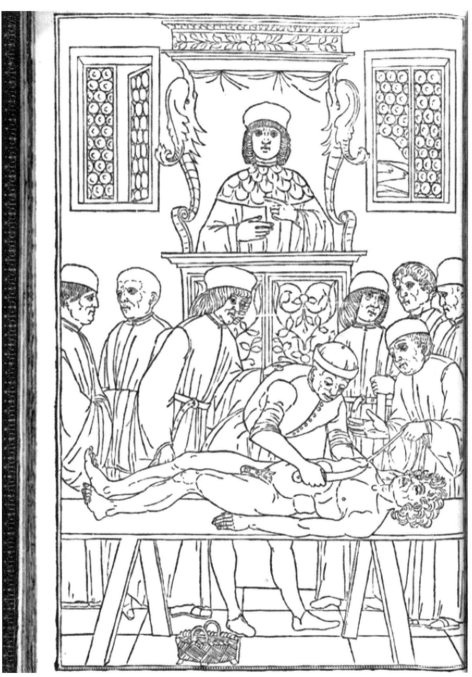

Figure 4.1. Illustration of an early anatomist (sitting) directing a dissection.
Source: S. DiMaio, F. Discepola, and R. F. Del Maestro, "Il Fasciculo di Medicina of 1493: Medical Culture through the Eyes of the Artist," Neurosurgery 58, no. 1 (January): 187–96, https://doi.org/10.1227/01.NEU.0000192382.37787.80. Courtesy of the National Library of Medicine

Vesalius redressed this practice, and one new anatomic finding after another reverberated as he corrected countless Galenic errors with great relish. Modern medical science had taken shape, even though it still was restricted to the study of the body from the neck down.

Interestingly, art played a crucial role in the explosion that launched the Scientific Revolution.[43] Vesalius's acquaintance with illustrator Johan van Calcar proved opportune for advancing the science of anatomy. Van Calcar, student of the renowned Venetian painter Titian, made brilliant and detailed woodcuts of Vesalius's early dissections—masterpieces unrivaled in detail (see figure 4.2).[44] Although Vesalius ignored crediting them, scholars generally agree that van Calcar and probably other students of Titian created the illustrations that set Vesalius's book apart, helping establish him as the preeminent anatomist and scientist of his day.[45]

The advantageous merging of art and science generated the exquisite, expensive publication of the *Fabrica*. Soon famous throughout Europe, the *Fabrica* ensured widespread circulation and promulgation of the new science; many called it the "greatest book in medicine."[46] Through this book, Vesalius inaugurated a new wave of scientific medicine, breaking the church's one-thousand-year stranglehold that had so impeded scientific progress.[47]

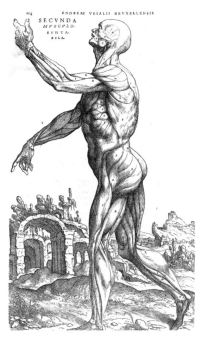

Figure 4.2.   Illustration from the *Fabrica*, attributed to Johan van Calcar.
Courtesy of Allard Pierson Heritage Collections, University of Amsterdam

The publication of Vesalius's *Fabrica* and the interest it spawned also contributed to a series of influential artworks depicting anatomical dissections—further merging the disciplines of art and science. Even though Pope Clement's decree permitted dissections, such events were few and far between. Therefore, when a physician had the opportunity to dissect a corpse, the occasion was unparalleled as a teaching tool, so students, other doctors, scientists, and even the public would pay a handsome sum to attend, as reported by historian-anatomist Sanjib Ghosh.[48]

Whose bodies did they dissect? Criminals. Once the spectacle of a public hanging had concluded, a new one took its place—dissecting the corpse. Dissections became exceptionally popular—as much entertainment for the community as education for clinicians.[49] They even led to the making of two of the Renaissance's greatest works of art. In Amsterdam on the last day of January 1632, authorities convicted Aris Kindt, known more commonly as Aris the Kid, for stealing a coat. They hanged him in the public square.[50] Dr. Nicolaes Tulp then proceeded to dissect the corpse before several students and colleagues—including a young, relatively unknown painter commissioned by the local surgeon's guild to record the unique event for posterity. The painter, twenty-six-year-old Rembrandt Harmenszoon van Rijn, later known simply as Rembrandt, painted his first tour de force of Renaissance art: *The Anatomy Lesson of Dr. Tulp*, a work that established his reputation as a master (see figure 4.3).[51] Posterity indeed.

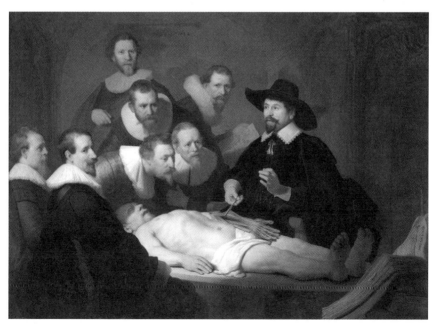

Figure 4.3.   Rembrandt van Rijn, *The Anatomy Lesson of Dr Nicolaes Tulp,* **1632.** *Courtesy of Mauritshuis, the Hague, Netherlands*

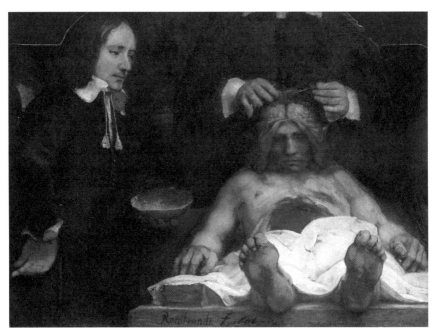

Figure 4.4. Rembrandt van Rijn, *The Anatomy Lesson of Dr. Deijman*, 1656. *Courtesy Amsterdam Museum; photo Amsterdam Museum*

Twenty-four years later, in 1656, Rembrandt painted *The Anatomy Lesson of Dr. Deijman*, depicting a brain dissection (see figure 4.4).[52] Dr. Jan Deijman replaced Dr. Tulp when the latter retired. When the authorities hanged criminal Joris Fonteijn as a thief, Dr. Deijman arranged for a public dissection that lasted three days, drawing hundreds of spectators. With both physicians and the public in attendance, Dr. Deijman opened Fonteijn's skull and dissected his brain, while Rembrandt documented the scene in another masterful, if macabre, portrait. Although Rembrandt depicted the brain attached to the body, likely for artistic impact, this was an exception. The old practice of separating the head from the body remained the predominant practice, and brain dissection was still rare, due to the church's influence.

Vesalius introduced another idea to medicine that was of equal impact to his study of anatomy but one often overlooked. He employed the kind of research methods that would guide and spur efforts by later scientists down to today. Going well beyond Hippocratic and Galenic scientific methods, this new technique entailed careful, firsthand observations of anatomic details; multiple observations in different corpses to identify variations in anatomic structures; and detailed recording of his findings—all devoid of Galen's church-based interpretations.[53] An objective, unemotional attitude complemented a focus on discovery and drawing conclusions that could be applied elsewhere based on what an individual observes.[54] A new atmosphere of inquiry emerged as Vesalius set the science of medicine on a solid foundation. The ancient authority of Galen was eradicated.[55]

Scientific Understanding Forges Ahead

The work of Vesalius and many subsequent scientists set the stage for modern medical science. Their discoveries in anatomy and physiology, as well as the scientific method itself, led to advances over the ensuing decades in gross anatomy, microscopic anatomy (histology), physiology, chemistry, and pathology (autopsy evaluation of diseases). Burgeoning numbers of scientists expanded previous findings and further contributed to the eventual understanding of the body as a hydraulic system of pipes and vessels—a mechanical system, a view still common today.[56] Furthermore, in advancing a mechanistic approach, these scientists addressed questions of how (How does the heart work?) rather than why (Why does the heart work?)—the latter still the church's province. This scientific understanding of body structure and function began to match that of escalating successes elsewhere in the more general Scientific Revolution in mathematics and physics.[57]

The modern focus on the physical body had sprung to life, though not yet incorporating patient care.[58] The specter of reductionism—explaining the whole person merely through understanding their individual physical body parts—loomed ominously. But for the present, clinical practitioners continued to incorporate the soul—or mind—in their treatment of patients.[59] They would not embrace the mind-body split until the early 1800s in Europe and the late 1800s in the United States.

CHAPTER 5

A Seventeenth-Century Philosophy Completes the Mind-Body Split

The Catholic Church's banning the head from human dissections in the sixteenth century played an important role in initiating the separation of mind and body. However, this split would become permanently entrenched in the seventeenth century, when powerful philosophical and theoretical thinkers, beginning with René Descartes, came to the fore. These thinkers formalized the idea that the sciences should concentrate exclusively on the physical and mechanical features of humankind. This new theory further steered anatomists, physiologists, and other scientists toward viewing the body as their domain while leaving the mind to the church.

This philosophy was the death knell for humanity in medical science, supplanting more than two millennia of holistic ideas that linked the mind and body. Scientists' sole interest in the body progressively embedded itself throughout the field of medicine over the ensuing centuries. Extraordinary advances followed, leading to the modern, disease-based medicine. But the mind-body split also had its downside: Avoiding psychological and social elements inflicted chaos on mental health care and other areas of medicine where the personal, emotional, and social features of patients were important.

My proposal is that, over the last four centuries, the medical profession has so firmly embraced the concept of mind-body separation that issues of the mind no longer fully register with medical thinkers; in fact, many believe that such mental concerns simply do not apply in medicine. Thus, mental health and other psychosocial dimensions now lie fallow in the "subconscious" of medical leaders and practitioners. This could explain medicine's seeming blind spot that almost completely ignores care for those with mental suffering. The mind and its emotions simply make no sense to the medical profession—such psychological concerns reside outside medicine's purview. But this creates a problem: To successfully provide care today for mental illnesses and chronic diseases, medicine must recognize the vast unseen landscape of the mind. As I explain in later chapters, because it's so ingrained and inaccessible in its subconscious, I believe medicine cannot achieve this goal without external pressure from the public and its politicians.

Note: I use the term *subconscious* as a metaphor.[1] Although familiar to many readers, this is not a standard term used in psychology, psychiatry, and psychoanalysis. The meaning I intend is a subliminal or hidden force that pushes medicine to act in ways it isn't fully aware of, such as diminishing mental health and other mind-related issues.

Descartes's Philosophical Theory Guides the Scientific Revolution

Most scholars consider René Descartes (1596–1650) the philosopher who most prominently influenced modern medicine by rejecting the mind to focus on bodily disease.[2] (See appendix A for an overview of how the mind-body split evolved.) Born in France, Descartes was a mathematician; scientist; and most importantly, a renowned philosopher. He made his greatest impact through his fascination with anatomy. According to historian Roy Porter and psychiatrist-philosopher Mark Sullivan, Descartes viewed the study of the human body—not the new physics or mathematics, which also became prominent during the Scientific Revolution—as the centerpiece of his natural science philosophy.[3] Although Descartes was not the first to address the mind-body dichotomy, most scholars agree that he played the key role in establishing a precedent for other philosophical influences that led to medicine's eventual approach, concentrating on the physical body and its diseases.[4]

Descartes posited that the soul (res cogitans: a thinking thing) was irrevocably separate from the body (res extensa: an extended thing) and that the two rarely—if ever—interacted. His celebrated phrase, "*Cogito, ergo sum*" (I think, therefore I am), reflected his fundamental idea that the mind (the soul) had immediate access to innate ideas because the mind existed independently of the body and its senses.[5] Descartes contrasted this to knowledge about the body, which took place slowly through the senses, such as seeing, hearing, or tasting. This basic concept rendered the mind and soul immune to corrupting outside influences—in a sense, immortalizing them.[6] Descartes had thus established the soul's eternal safety and—hoping to please the powerful Catholic Church—argued that scientific inquiry should center on the body and its external world, investigating its physical mechanisms, as Vesalius had begun and others continued. This idea appealed to the church and scientific communities alike. Descartes's soul thus makes room for religion and human dignity but at considerable cost to society; it essentially authorizes the mind-body dichotomy. Some go so far as to say that Descartes's philosophy represents a grand historic compromise with the church, allowing medical science to define the body, as long as it left the mind and soul to the church.[7]

Descartes laid the groundwork for two equally prominent philosophers who would extend and reinforce the mind-body duality: Thomas Hobbes and John Locke. The first, British philosopher Thomas Hobbes (1588–1679), was an atheist, so unlike Descartes, he felt little need to please the church. In fact, Hobbes dismissed the subjective mind altogether, denying the reality of anything but objective, concrete matter, such as the body.[8] He regarded the universe as a continuum of matter devoid of spirit.

Soon after Descartes's death, a second philosopher, John Locke (1632–1704), emerged, whose impact many view as even more lasting and consequential.[9] Locke was a revered physician; writer (famed for his *Two Treatises of Government*); and, later in life, philosopher. He also rejected Descartes's concept of innate ideas as unnecessary and simply ignored the troublesome question of how the mind interacts with the body.[10] Like Descartes, Locke consigned the mind and soul to the church. A profound influence on the growing cadre of new scientists, Locke focused on physical causes or mechanisms to explain *how* the body worked. (The more speculative *why*, a question regarding the mind or soul, he left to the church.[11]) He believed, as Descartes had, that studying anatomy and physiology rather than mathematics or physics yielded the best scientific guidance for understanding humankind's interaction with the world.[12]

The mind-body dichotomy held major implications for present-day practitioners. First, one could only experience the mind/soul from the inside, making it impossible to examine the mind and its mental disorders. Next, this dichotomy would influence modern medicine's penchant for objectivity; the clinician had to investigate the body from the outside as an object—not viewing the patient as a living, feeling person—and to view the patient in the same objective way that multiple viewers of a body would see it.[13]

By the late seventeenth century, medical science centered almost entirely on the bodily features of human beings. Technological developments spurred the basic scientific advances that continued into the eighteenth century, spreading well beyond the anatomy depicted by Vesalius to physiology, chemistry, microscopic anatomy, and pathologic anatomy.[14]

The revolution at this point, however, had involved just research in these basic medical sciences. While such research was significant to the development of science, it had not directly improved patients' conditions and did not influence clinical practice. Although practitioners of the sixteenth through the eighteenth centuries finally shelved Galen's ideas, which they now considered a mockery of medicine, they turned back to Hippocrates for direction and continued to view the mind and body as one. However, this also meant practitioners still interpreted symptoms as punishment from God—a belief held by Galen and the ancient Greeks alike.[15] In addition, they continued to believe that an imbalance of the four humors (blood, phlegm, yellow bile, and black bile) represented disease, and they still classified each disease by its own collection of symptoms.[16] This necessitated taking careful histories of both a patient's personal issues and physical symptoms; meanwhile they performed only a cursory physical examination, if they did so at all. But new discoveries on the horizon spelled the end of this ancient, Hippocratic approach to clinical medicine.

Evolution of Clinical Medicine

A concentration on the objective, definable features of the physical body would now emerge, as clinicians renounced patients' subjective, personal attributes. Human dissections again played a key role in producing the shift from Hippocratic medicine. In the mid- to late eighteenth centuries, autopsy findings introduced the mind-body duality into clinical medicine.[17] By the early nineteenth century, French medical science had launched the new clinical direction in medicine and its hospitals. The influence of this development soon spread widely throughout England, Austria, and Germany, arriving in America in the late nineteenth century.[18]

AUTOPSIES INITIATE THE BIRTH OF
MODERN CLINICAL MEDICINE

Autopsies prompted eighteenth-century clinicians to adopt a radical new belief: that the abnormal organs and tissues they discovered represented the diseases that caused these patients' deaths. Doctors further deduced that the diseased structures caused the patients' symptoms—a concept that replaced the two-millennia-old belief that symptoms stemmed from an imbalance in the four humors and represented punishment for one's sins. The shift would forever alter clinicians' understanding of disease and their approach to patients. Modern, scientific clinical care had begun.

Giovanni Battista Morgagni (1682–1771), often considered the "father of anatomic pathology," launched this revolution in medical reasoning, according to physician and writer Sherwin Nuland.[19] Morgagni's famous book *De sedibus et causis morborum per anatomen indagatis* (*On the Seats and Causes of Diseases Investigated through Anatomy*), posited that abnormal autopsy findings, such as an inflamed lung or a swollen liver, represented the disease and produced its symptoms, such as pain upon breathing or upper-right-sided abdominal pain, respectively.[20] The idea of linking symptoms to abnormal organs seen at autopsy wasn't new, but Morgagni, a clinician, systematized the concept, hoping to guide doctors to better diagnoses.[21] He painstakingly conducted seven hundred autopsies over his lifetime and then correlated abnormal findings with patients' symptoms, which he obtained from their clinical records.[22] However, medicine at this early point had not yet identified actual causes of any diseases; this would require more specific knowledge that would later evolve in clinical medicine, particularly in chemistry, microscopy, and bacteriology.[23]

The following is one of Morgagni's shorter case reports of a young woman who died of severe inflammation involving the lining of the heart (pericardium), which accounts for the profusion of fluid he observed at the autopsy.[24] Today's more advanced knowledge and expertise would likely identify her condition with greater specificity: A good modern guess is that tuberculosis or some other infection caused the inflammation and, in turn, the fluid:

Case Report

A maiden fifteen years of age was affected with acute fever, but she was more particularly distressed from excruciating pain in the head. About the tenth day the febrile symptoms were mitigated; but a few days afterwards, in addition to the fever, she experienced considerable thirst, and difficulty of breathing, accompanied with pain in the left side of the chest. The dyspnea (shortness of breath) and pain in the chest became increasingly oppressive within a few days, and she expired.

Dissection. The lungs were healthy, but the left cavity of the chest was full of serum (fluid), in which some concretions floated, which bore a resemblance to hardened albumen. The right cavity likewise contained a redundance of serous fluid, but it was small in quantity. The pericardium was replete with fluid, which was somewhat thicker than that which occupied the thorax; and the surface of the heart was slightly eroded.

At the end of the century, François Bichat (1771–1802) followed Morgagni in the study of autopsy findings, making notable discoveries regarding the significance of tissues.[25] He found that the body consisted of twenty-one separate tissues, such as arteries, muscle, mucous membrane linings, nerves, glands, and bone. This greatly expanded on Morgagni's findings: Bichat showed that diseases occurred in the tissues of an organ rather than the whole organ itself.[26] (It would be another fifty years before Rudolf Virchow [1821–1902] established that cellular disorders caused the tissue and organ changes of disease.[27]) For those still unconvinced, philosopher Michel Foucault (1926–1984) reported that Bichat suggested they simply "open up a few corpses."[28] Bichat's findings raised the bar for making more precise disease diagnoses from abnormalities of tissues observed at autopsies; such tissues included hardened coronary arteries causing a "heart attack"; thin, dilated heart muscle causing "heart failure"; and inflammation of the heart's outside lining (pericardium) causing "pericarditis." It was no longer satisfactory to make a simple diagnosis of "heart disease."

In sum, the revolutionary idea of associating symptoms with autopsy findings had begun; this concept, termed *clinical-pathological correlation*, flourishes to this day in clinical medicine.[29] That is, physical symptoms are clues to an underlying physical disease.

THE "GAZE" OF CLINICAL CARE SHIFTS

Foucault captured this revolutionary morphing to clinical pathological correlation in his classic *The Birth of the Clinic: An Archeology of Medical Perception*.[30] He highlighted that the physician's "gaze" had repositioned—no longer viewing symptoms as punishment from God or stemming from humoral imbalances but reflecting objectively identifiable disease. Due to the dramatic new findings and concepts of Morgagni and Bichat, clinicians rapidly changed their focus: Now they looked to identify symptoms suggesting an underlying disease to be found at autopsy. Unfortunately, embracing this direction also had a downside that plagues medicine to this day. The new perspective meant abandoning a Hippocratic, holistic view and led to an impersonal understanding of the patient.

Two changes reoriented clinicians. First, physicians continued to conduct detailed questioning but now only regarding bodily symptoms that suggested an underlying disease; they excluded the patient's personal experience of illness.[31] Physician and philosopher Mark Sullivan indicates that clinicians no longer asked a patient about his or her job, family, or emotions, believing the psychosocial components superfluous.[32] Instead of inquiring, "How are you doing?" or "How did you feel about that?" they would simply ask, "Where is the pain located, when did it begin, any nausea or vomiting?" or "Is there a fever or cough?" or "Did you see blood?" In a second change, while doctors intensively questioned the patient, they placed even more value on the physical examination: for example, palpating an enlarged liver or hearing a telltale heart sound.[33] They believed, often correctly, that such abnormal examination findings foretold a disease they might discover at autopsy.[34] In sum, the patient became nothing but a mystery to solve for the presence of a disease—a common view for modern clinicians. Questioning patients regarding symptoms and the physical examination became more important than the actual person.

Following the discoveries of Morgagni and Bichat, technical advances in microscopy and chemistry promoted the spread of the new clinical revolution, particularly those of Virchow.[35] Viewing human tissue through the microscope further refined understanding of diseases identified at autopsy.[36] For example, for the first time, physicians could see thousands of cancerous cells in tissues that explained the large growths seen at autopsy. They also saw microscopic scarring (cirrhosis) in tissue removed from the livers of alcohol abusers that explained the liver's shrunken, whitened autopsy appearance.[37] New knowledge in chemistry enabled additional understanding of diseases where scientists observed no abnormalities at autopsy or under the microscope; for example, high blood sugars in diabetes.[38] With such advances, the modern-day belief emerged that every disease possessed some demonstrably visible or microscopic defect in body structure or altered chemistry—and that such defects linked to each disease were unique.[39]

THE LEGACY OF CLINICAL-PATHOLOGICAL CORRELATION

The course set by Morgagni and Bichat continues to this day. Indeed, making clinical-pathological correlations—linking symptoms and physical examination findings to an underlying disease—is the holy grail of the modern disease-oriented physician. To make such links, the doctor continues to identify the various constellations of symptoms and physical exam findings that may offer clues to underlying diseases.[40] Medicine's understanding of disease diagnoses continues to progress through consideration of symptoms. In fact, present-day care now regards symptoms more valuable than physical exam findings in making diagnoses.[41]

Today the clinician has more tools at his or her disposal than ever before. Many laboratory and other tests now are available to complement the diagnostic accuracy of symptoms.[42] And to confirm the presence of a disease, the modern clinician also has many means beyond autopsy findings; such means range from genetic testing and taking a biopsy sample from tissue suspected as diseased to performing various types of radiographic imaging and blood testing.

What explains the pervasiveness of clinical-pathological correlation?[43] Given medical educators' predisposition toward physical diseases, they teach clinical-pathological correlation as the centerpiece of medical students' education. Students in the first two years learn what "normal" looks like by taking courses in anatomy and histology (microscopic anatomy). Then they learn about deviations from normal—the gross (visible without a microscope) and microscopic autopsy findings of virtually all diseases (pathology). In the last two clinical years, students integrate this knowledge of diseases with real patient experiences. They learn the symptom, physical exam, and testing features of literally hundreds of patients with various diseases, such as heart attacks, emphysema, appendicitis, colon cancer, gallstones, and many others.

An example of the central role clinical-pathological correlation in modern medicine shows up in the world's most prominent medical journal, the *New England Journal of Medicine*. The journal often devotes a portion of its publication to solving a disease mystery in a format called a clinical-pathological conference, familiar to all students as the CPC.[44] The organizers of the CPC present a deceased patient's symptoms, physical examination, and laboratory data to a seasoned clinician, who does not yet know the diagnosis; they select a difficult-to-diagnose patient, one with an unusual disease or an infrequent presentation of a common disease.[45] The clinician eruditely discusses the information before a large audience of faculty and learners and then offers the disease diagnosis he or she believes explains the patient's problem. How do attendees know whether the clinician solved the mystery correctly? The pathologist confirms or refutes the clinician's diagnosis with "hard data" from an autopsy or other definitive sources of disease information, such as a biopsy, genetic testing, or radiographic imaging. Not surprisingly, no one mentions "soft data" regarding the patient's personal concerns, mental health, or emotions.

FAST-FORWARDING TO THE PRESENT

While diagnoses improved as clinicians gained a better understanding of diseases, treatment lagged. In truth, from the eighteenth through the early twentieth centuries, therapy created mostly harm. For example, in addition to prescribing dangerous medications for constipation and toxic mercury as an antiseptic, they continued the practice—since Hippocratic times—of bloodletting or application of as many as fifty leeches as ways to extract blood in attempts to rebalance the four humors.

It will no doubt unsettle American and Canadian physicians to learn that their most revered clinician, William Osler, advocated bloodletting.[46] From the 1912 edition of his 1892 textbook, he writes, "Pneumonia is one of the diseases in which a timely venesection may save life. . . . The abstraction of from twenty to thirty ounces of blood is in every way beneficial."[47] Voltaire's (1694–1778) keen insight portrayed the essence of clinical care in the eighteenth century, which applied in the nineteenth, as well: "Doctors are men who prescribe medicine of which they know little to cure diseases of which they know less in human beings of which they know nothing."[48]

Unhappily, doctors lacked an effective pharmacological arsenal until the late nineteenth and early twentieth centuries.[49] The first treatment advances came from a surprising source in the late 1800s. The chemical industry—rather than scientists—produced many useful therapeutic agents: aspirin and opium alkaloids for pain, chloral hydrate for sleep, sulphonal for anxiety, nitroglycerin for heart disease, salvarsan (an arsenic product) for syphilis, quinine for malaria, and diphtheria antitoxin.[50] Finally, the clinician had an effective therapeutic reach and could offer more than just a careful clinical evaluation and a diagnosis. But progress had only begun.

Antibiotics arrived with sulfa drugs—the first medications to treat bacterial infections—in 1935, followed shortly by an even more powerful antibiotic, penicillin.[51] The floodgates soon opened with a cornucopia of successes, controlling and curing many different types of infections: for example, abscesses, strep throat, pneumonia, and diarrhea. Over the next several decades, massive proliferation of these and other new drugs ensued. In time, they controlled and sometimes eradicated most acute infectious diseases, the scourges of the day.

The discovery of anesthesia and improved surgical techniques also fostered improvements previously unimagined, reports surgeon-historian David Schneider.[52] For example, a physician could now put a patient to sleep with newly discovered ether or chloroform and pull a tooth, fix a fracture, or even amputate a limb without that person enduring the excruciating, devastating pain of surgery. Before they had performed such procedures on conscious patients—drugged only with alcohol.[53]

Disease-oriented medicine rapidly reached its pinnacle by the mid- and late twentieth century. Using antibiotics, surgery, and especially emerging public health measures to combat epidemics, an increasingly scientific medical profession could now treat and control and even, in many instances, cure former death warrants, such as pneumonia, tonsillitis, tuberculosis, rheumatic fever, erysipelas, typhoid fever, and diphtheria. Patients now lived where their ancestors had succumbed to disease only a short time before.

Over time, with the support of escalating successes and new research findings, disease-oriented medicine became more complex; specialization followed, which fostered greater achievement but an increasingly narrow focus on bodily disease. Today, fewer than one-half of clinicians attend to the whole patient in primary care.[54] Instead, the majority specialize in body parts or functions, requiring patients to see an array of clinicians, each restricted to a particular part and its disorders.

From the standpoint of life survival, however, the focus on the body paid off in spades. According to the Centers for Disease Control and Prevention and others, Americans' life span doubled from forty years of age in 1900 to nearly eighty by 2014 thanks to numerous continuing advances in public health measures and in treatment of such diseases as polio, heart disease, cancer, and AIDS.[55] To appreciate the enormity of this metamorphosis, recall that little actual treatment progress had taken place since the time of Hippocrates more than two millennia ago. Then in the twentieth century, human life span doubled within about one hundred years. What about that for progress, due to the Scientific Revolution's focus on physical illness, which triggered effective diagnosis and treatment efforts to control disease?[56]

Despite these impressive figures, recent data from the prestigious National Academy of Sciences, Engineering, and Medicine show a reduction in life expectancy from 2015 to 2017 related to an increase in deaths in twenty-five to sixty-four-year-olds. Psychosocially based problems caused most of the deaths: substance abuse, suicide, and lifestyle diseases; more recently, the coronavirus pandemic caused the life expectancy statistics to dip further by 2021, with only an incomplete recovery by 2022.[57]

Origin of US Medical Education

Medical schools' failure to prepare US physicians for mental health took place in parallel with the clinical revolution developing in America in the late nineteenth century. By this time, many thousands of American doctors had studied in the medical centers of Europe, where they imported the radical new precept of clinical-pathological correlation to identify physical diseases.[58] They also brought technical advances, such as the stethoscope, and the European tradition that care occurred in the hospital, the clinician's "laboratory."[59]

Medical historian Roy Porter relates that, in 1889, the Johns Hopkins Hospital became the first American institution to embody the clinical ideas developed in Europe.[60] Hopkins pioneered the teaching of these concepts from overseas that would enter US medical education. Over the next quarter century, Hopkins's model of objective clinical care based on clinical-pathological correlation—along with rigorous experimental research—replaced the voluminous hodgepodge of one- to two-year proprietary schools in this country. Prescientific relics, such as bloodletting, leeches, and purgatives, finally disappeared, and the superior European approach quickly took hold.

To operationalize this, the American Medical Association commissioned the Carnegie Foundation and Abraham Flexner (1866–1959) to evaluate American education. The Flexner Report of 1910 determined the content of modern medical education, and it still shapes US health care today.[61] Its guidance led authorities to require that medical schools adopt the Hopkins model of much longer, more rigorous teaching that included actual supervised experiences with diseased patients.[62] Authorities forced most schools to close because they could not uphold the new standard.[63]

The Flexner Report ensured that the explosion of medical schools during this time would teach only disease based medicine and that the proliferation of hospitals would focus almost exclusively on physical disorders.[64] Meanwhile, also reflecting European practices, medical school curricular requirements for psychiatry were miniscule and have evolved little—if any—in more than one hundred years.[65] The steamrolling European influence prevailed uncontested, allowing no opportunity to introduce any alternative.

Keep the Flexner Report in mind; I return to it in the final chapter.

What Happened to the Mind and Mental Illness?

Although the medical profession shunned mental illness almost completely until the nineteenth century, mental disorders did not disappear by any means. Up to the late eighteenth century, most care took place in patients' homes and through community resources.[66] More severe disorders received help at church-based medieval hospitals, monasteries, and religious houses.[67] As the new scientific medicine expanded, however, its principles spilled over to mental illnesses, especially efforts to tie symptoms of mental disorders to an underlying brain disease. A good model for this existed in the striking autopsy abnormalities seen in the brains of patients who died of general paresis of the insane, the devastating dementia of neurosyphilis. However, clinicians had found no similar telltale autopsy abnormalities in other recognized mental disorders of this time, such as those labeled melancholia, mania, idiocy, and other types of dementia.[68]

In a secular shift, the new disease orientation opened the door for physicians to take charge of mental care institutions, initially called "lunatic asylums." In the United States, a corps of specialists slowly materialized from the physicians running the asylums, presaging the birth of psychiatry as a discipline. By the mid-nineteenth century, the small field of psychiatry had evolved into a formal organization, the Association of Medical Superintendents of American Institutions for the Insane. They published their own scientific journal, the *American Journal of Insanity*, now the prestigious *American Journal of Psychiatry*.[69]

Early psychiatric hospitals terrified doctors, as well as patients, and needed radical improvement. Asylum care, noteworthy also for its filthiness, had infamously employed punitive conditions, including prolonged isolation, chain restraints, corporal punishment, straitjackets, handcuffs, and electric shock treatment.

Revolted by such conditions, the new psychiatric hospitals substituted what they called "moral treatment" for old asylum care. This return to Hippocratic traditions placed the patient in his or her psychological, emotional, and social realms foremost. However, hospitals had no choice but to utilize the same prescientific treatments for actual diseases customary at this time, such as bloodletting and leeches. And despite these institutions' noble intent, abuses continued into the second half of the nineteenth century. Nonetheless, the asylum movement accelerated and provided care for more and more patients over time.[70]

While the asylums made little positive impact on patients' actual mental health, psychiatry itself made significant progress in another direction. With increasing numbers of patients admitted, psychiatrists conducted extensive investigations to generate better understanding of mental disorders and improve their classifications.[71] Indeed, they identified such conditions as epilepsy and Down syndrome and no longer labeled them as mental illnesses.

The academic foundations of psychiatry continued to evolve, culminating by the late nineteenth century with such illustrious leaders as Emil Kraepelin (1856–1926) and Sigmund Freud (1856–1939).[72] Psychiatrists also continued to consider the broader psychological and social dimensions as important, but they continued to believe in the idea of physical disease as the cause of psychological disorders, despite an absence of evidence.

By the early twentieth century, only the tiny field of psychiatry assumed responsibility for mental health. Despite continued beliefs that disease caused mental illness, psychiatry's attention to psychological and social interests in the early and mid-1900s generated some hope for retaining a person-centered, humane focus in mental health. Nobel laureate and psychiatrist-neuroscientist Eric Kandel indicates that, as neuroscience matured, it has discarded or modified many of Freud's ideas. However, Freud's articulation of the unconscious and its impact on understanding patients' personal characteristics remains monumentally important, guiding psychology to this day.[73] Freud's concept of listening carefully to the patient while facilitating the flow of conversation also survives in the field of patient-centered interviewing.

The key role of mental features got more support when World Wars I and II revealed a surprising chink in the armor of disease-oriented medicine. The wars brought widespread recognition that neither clinicians nor patients could explain certain bodily symptoms as a result of an injury or disease.[74] Soldiers were coming home with a condition labeled "traumatic war neuroses" or "shell shock": symptoms developed when a soldier experienced an enemy attack that killed or severely harmed his comrades, while the soldier himself survived with minimal or no harm. Physicians understood the anxiety of a near-miss but not the terribly persisting and disabling physical symptoms, for which they would have puzzled, "But there's nothing wrong." Recognized now as post-traumatic stress disorder, the condition causes patients to experience the same unexplained symptoms, such as protracted pain, fatigue, dizziness, and insomnia.[75] Clinicians now recognize that the symptoms can follow severe stressors of many types: for example, sexual, corporal, and psychological abuse. Disease-based experts cannot explain the physical symptoms—an anomaly that doesn't fit into the present disease-only theoretical model. Therefore, it's most likely that today's patients—the prime example, sufferers of chronic pain—will receive ineffective treatment.

Despite its promising beginning, psychiatry took a turn backward as the twentieth century wore on. Many scholars lament that concerns for patients' psychological and social issues now faded out of sight.[76] Psychiatry itself fell further prey to its long-term hope of finding a brain disease to explain mental disorders. This is not entirely surprising because scientific knowledge of the brain and its functions had advanced by leaps and bounds.[77]

Then, with the development of new drugs, psychiatry increasingly concentrated on physical and chemical explanations for disorders, a trend that persists to this day. The discovery of lithium in 1948 and chlorpromazine (Thorazine) in 1952 initiated this direction. These drugs revolutionized treatment for bipolar disorder (then called manic depression) and schizophrenia, respectively.[78] The discovery of the benzodiazepines, Valium the prototype, followed soon after.[79] These breakthroughs launched the psychopharmacological approach that has characterized clinical psychiatry ever since.[80]

Thomas Insel, a clinical and research psychiatrist and former director of the National Institute of Mental Health, and others repeatedly spotlight the futility of modern psychiatry's approach with one fact: They have made no significant impact on care for mental disorders in the last twenty-five years.[81] Indeed, in his new book *Healing: Our Path from Mental Illness to Mental Health*, Insel labels poor mental health care a human rights issue. Nevertheless, psychiatry now continues to rely heavily on drugs, paradoxically discarding its crucial early advances of listening carefully to the patient and seeking to understand their psychological issues.[82]

Why Cartesian Theory Is Important

Few in medicine today question Descartes's theory separating the mind from the body—sweeping aside its limitations that brought about the ongoing crisis in mental illness and chronic disease.[83] The grave consequences of this enduring philosophy clearly illustrate a disconnect between how the medical profession performs and what the public actually needs.[84] The resulting adverse outcomes are so severe and so obvious that some label the theory of mind-body duality as apocryphal— a mythical concept that falls far from the truth yet continues to be used.[85] Medicine plows ahead, facts aside, by following an effete philosophy.[86]

The power of any theory resides in establishing the foundation for constructing knowledge—and thereby establishing how scientists generate scientific progress. Theory dictates how scientists and physicians conduct research, think about their discipline, care for their patients, and teach their students.[87] Once scientists adopt a guiding philosophy, few ever reconsider how it operates; it simply becomes automatic. This thinking also persists because educators indoctrinate students with it.[88] Most scientists don't even recognize that theory undergirds their research methods. While familiar scientific methods, such as randomized controlled trials, define *how* they conduct studies, famous scientist-philosopher Karl Popper and others emphasize that it is scientific theory that determines *what* research ideas scientists will examine.[89]

The following study is an example of how Descartes's model influences researchers to focus their work on physical disease. My Michigan State group reviewed the literature to see how well medical research has incorporated "patient-centeredness," a measure of relevant psychosocial and mental information obtained from patients. We found extraordinarily telling results. Out of 327,219 randomized controlled trials, medicine's most powerful research method, conducted by 2010, only 1,475 studies (0.5 percent) even mentioned being patient-centered.[90] This means that 99.5 percent of studies cannot inform the most important psychological, social, and emotional attributes of a patient's life.

Scientific Revolution philosophers were conscious of what they advocated. But medical leaders and practitioners and the public simply followed their lead—without giving much thought, if any, to an alternative. And mind-related topics, such as mental health, progressively sank into their subconscious recesses. Soon psychological issues and mental illnesses disappeared, along with medicine's ancient Hippocratic heritage and medicine's soul.

Who's at Fault?

Should you hold Descartes responsible for medicine ignoring psychosocial concerns? Many scholars do.[91] On the contrary, I believe that the medical and scientific communities and the public should, in fact, commend Descartes. The blame lies elsewhere.

Descartes's contribution revolutionized medicine in a true paradigm shift from the concept of the four humors to that of clinical pathological correlation.[92] The new scientists, led by Descartes, demythologized the body and, over time, gave birth to modern scientific medicine. The advances that followed Descartes created the unrivaled disease benefits the public now accepts as routine—an auspicious beginning for modern health care that reached its zenith midway through the last century. Nevertheless, an unhappy side surfaced late in the last century, as well. Why? The public has experienced no parallel progress for integrating patients' psychological and social features into health care, though this time it is medicine, not the church, that bears responsibility.[93]

Don't blame Descartes: *It is modern medicine that deserves reproach because, following Descartes, medicine's theoretical and intellectual progress came to a halt.*

Since the Scientific Revolution, the profession has played out the admittedly productive disease hand while failing to incorporate mental illnesses and other psychosocial issues. In short, medicine remains irrationally hooked on the mind-body dichotomy, an idea that prevents it from incorporating psychosocial and mental health features into patients' care.[94]

Can medicine open its eyes to the dilemma and implement a modern theory? Ample precedents exist in science for progressing from one successful theory to an improved one, such as the path of Isaac Newton's (1642–1727) pioneering model in physics—an example from Descartes's own century. Later, in the twentieth century, Albert Einstein (1879–1955) and others transformed Newton's own standard-changing findings into the new physics without sacrificing Newton's seminal advances.[95]

What will medicine require to similarly grow and mature as a science? A new theory must build on Descartes's advances to continue medicine's progress in controlling diseases but, at the same time, incorporate the mind and mental issues.

CHAPTER 6

A Twenty-First-Century Systems View Integrates Mind and Body

Over the last century, a modern scientific theory has emerged to replace medicine's narrow focus on disease: a systems view of life. In their extensively detailed, seminal book *A Systems View of Life: A Unifying Vision*, Fritjof Capra and Pier Luigi Luisi lay out this new theory of science.[1] The philosophy they describe can furnish the theoretical basis for healing the mental health and chronic disease dilemma. I believe that implementing this view is paramount, not only for the health care purposes, but also for restoring medicine's soul, its humanity. In addition, I fear that not adopting a systems perspective jeopardizes medicine's status as a scientific discipline. Failure to take on this view would lead to further decline in both psychological and physical disease care and create massive increases in health care costs.

A Systems View

The systems view represents a new way of scientific thinking that provides an overarching bridge between the many scientific disciplines. It posits that the many component parts of any scientific subject interact so that they illustrate the big picture—the holistic representation of the subject.[2] Think of your family as a demonstration of how this works. Families consist of various members, typically parents and children, often grandparents, and perhaps an animal or two. Yet knowing a family requires more than adding up the facts about its members; it's understanding how they interact. A similar concept exists throughout all sciences. For instance, a cell is not defined by the very existence of the mitochondria, nucleus, and other parts but by how all these components work together. Indeed, Austrian systems biologist Paul Weiss (1898–1989) stated the famous systems axiom "The whole equals more than the sum of its parts."[3] This concept

73

equally applies in nonscientific contexts. A brief excerpt from a famous passage by the revered seventeenth-century English scholar, poet, and cleric John Donne (1572–1631) conveys the same message: "No man is an Iland, intire of it selfe; every man is a peece of the Continent, a part of the maine."[4]

In contrast to a systems view, Cartesian thinking would contend that knowledge of individual family members in isolation, without their interactions, would suffice to understand the family and its needs. Though common experience refutes this, the Cartesian view insists on this idea. This reasoning defies the basic systems concept that all parts within the whole are fundamentally interdependent; therefore, all must be considered.[5]

All the sciences initially followed the reductionistic ideas of the Scientific Revolution—reducing concepts to one or two elements while ignoring many others. Yet they all—except medicine—eventually discarded this mode of thinking to adopt a systems view. Dramatic benefits followed: for example, relativity and quantum theories in physics, cybernetics in mathematics and engineering, gestalt theory in psychology, complexity theory and fractal geometry in nonlinear systems, general systems theory in biology, information theory, and game theory.[6]

Much of the public undoubtedly view these theories as obscure, irrelevant to everyday existence; however, these theories have practical applications that bring them to life and underscore the importance of the new systems view. For example, consider the discoveries that led to victories by the Allied Forces in World War II.[7] Mathematics experts, led by Alan Turing (1912–1954), worked with Britain's secret code-breaking center at Bletchley Park to break the code of the German Enigma machine.[8] The principles Turing identified during this time, such as algorithm and computation, would become the basis of modern computing and artificial intelligence. Today most view Turing as the father of modern computing.[9] Meanwhile, experts in cybernetics—the science of control and communication in animals and the machine—contributed to the war effort by developing new gunnery systems for tracking and shooting down enemy aircraft; this gave the Allied Forces a real tactical advantage with much-needed dominance of the skies.[10]

After the war, the sciences continued to apply the systems view in an expanding range of domains. The cyberneticists employed it to demonstrate the neural mechanisms underlying mind functions—the workings of thinking and consciousness. Their efforts culminated in the science of cognition, which demonstrated an indisputable link between the brain and other body *structures* and the *process* of thinking. This laid the mind-body duality to rest scientifically and conceptually once and for all.[11] Systems scientists went on to bridge the gap from mathematics, engineering, and neuroscience to include the humanities, where Gregory Bateson (1904–1980) portrayed the mind as a systems phenomenon.

Taking this thinking even further, Bateson identified the clinical need for a systems strategy when working with troubled families—the advent of family therapy.[12] Modern ecology also evolved from a systems view of interaction between the population and the environment.[13]

I'll go way out on a limb and predict that, if medicine adopts the new systems view, the field will experience similar revolutionary changes. And these advances will be of equal magnitude to those achieved in physics, mathematics, ecology, and biology: for example, improving the lives of those millions currently suffering with unattended mental and chronic physical disorders, eliminating deaths from incorrectly prescribed medications and preventable suicides, and producing massive savings. Yet medicine alone among the scientific disciplines remains attached to Cartesian theoretical principles that no longer make sense today.

GENERAL SYSTEMS THEORY

General systems theory is the most appropriate systems view to orchestrate a new direction in medicine because it emerges from biology and the study of living organisms.[14] Preeminent biologists Ludwig von Bertalanffy (1901–1972) and Paul Weiss, along with many others, described this in the early twentieth century.[15]

The same concept of parts and whole forms the basis of general systems theory. This concept is illustrated in the hierarchy of natural systems in figure 6.1. Each system level progresses in complexity, starting at the bottom with subatomic particles; moving up to atoms, molecules, cells, tissues, organs, body systems, the individual, the family, the community, the society; until finally reaching the highest level, the cosmos.[16] Each level in the hierarchy is discrete and unique, with a structural and functional connection to the level above and below via continuous feedback loops, as lucidly portrayed by family physician and philosopher Howard Brody (1949–2024).

To depict a systems view, I earlier offered examples where many individual members act together to make up a family and several individual cell components interact to make up a cell. Similarly, multiple individual entities at any given level in the hierarchy of natural systems interact to form the next higher level. While various theories offer insight into how the parts interrelate to generate a new whole at any level, these parts interact in still difficult-to-understand, nonlinear ways to lead to the unique next level.[17] The parts exchange information differently at each level: for example, molecular interactions at the cellular level, cognition and perception at the individual person level, and social relations at the family level.

The Hierarchy of Natural Systems

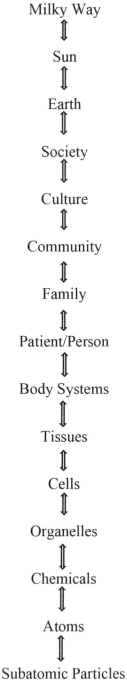

Milky Way

Sun

Earth

Society

Culture

Community

Family

Patient/Person

Body Systems

Tissues

Cells

Organelles

Chemicals

Atoms

Subatomic Particles

Figure 6.1.   Systems hierarchy

The many scientific disciplines, such as physics, medicine, psychology, and anthropology, fit into this hierarchy of systems; each discipline can include a range of levels, with the focus of the field falling at the centermost point. For example, considering the various levels in figure 6.1, a physicist would concentrate on subatomic particles, atoms, and chemicals; an anthropologist, on communities, culture, and society; and an astronomer, on the earth, sun, and Milky Way. So where does medicine fit? The biopsychosocial model provides the answer.

The Biopsychosocial Model

As a broad-based discipline, medicine spans several levels of the systems hierarchy. But the level at its center must be the individual for whom it provides care: the patient.[18] As a subset of general systems theory, the *biopsychosocial model* articulates how the biological (physical) and the social (environmental) levels relate to the patient (psychological) level. Figure 6.2 identifies the model's location within the systems hierarchy with the labels "bio-," "psycho-," and "social." Joining these elements together, with the patient at the center, clinicians have the biopsychosocial model as the systems view of medicine. While medicine's current guiding theory remains the biomedical, or disease-only, model, the biopsychosocial model incorporates physical diseases in the "bio" portion of the new model, so it retains the benefits of this dimension.

As a systems-based science, medicine must equally represent biological, psychological, and social components in research, teaching, and patient care. Only in this way can it adequately address its primary focus: the patient. A focus by the entire profession on any one of these three dimensions flouts general systems theory, as medicine now does by concentrating almost exclusively on the biological, or physical disease, level. Put another way, each individual biopsychosocial level is necessary but not sufficient to explain the patient's health status. Especially crucial is studying interactions both within levels and between levels, according to Robert Ader (1932–2011), psychologist, researcher, and discoverer of the link between the brain and the immunological system.[19]

Of course, some individual professionals within medicine may focus on one subset of these levels; the psychologist will naturally concentrate at the patient level; the cell biologist, below that level; and the anthropologist, above that at the social level. Also, the relevant balances of biopsychosocial components may vary for individual patients at any given time.

The Biopsychosocial Model within the Systems Hierarchy

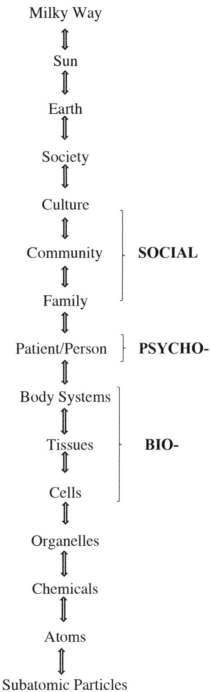

Figure 6.2.   Biopsychosocial model

Provenance of the Biopsychosocial Model and Its Problems

In 1977, George Libman Engel (1913–1999) at the University of Rochester incorporated medicine into general systems theory by articulating the biopsychosocial model. Engel based it on his wide-ranging experiences in medicine, psychoanalysis, and psychiatry and aimed to enhance the humanistic, as well as scientific, status of medicine.[20] As you know, Dr. Engel played a key role in my career as a friend, mentor, and colleague. I know I'm biased, but I think many will agree that he will go down in history as a giant of twentieth-century medicine.[21] (Appendix A identifies the Engel model's crucial place in the mind-body dichotomy's history.)

Medical schools rapidly embraced the biopsychosocial model in their teaching and mission statements alike. Following the initial excitement, however, the model showed limited overall impact on medicine's patient care and research—and received mostly lip service.[22] So what was the problem? After all, it provided the necessary theoretical backing required to improve mental health and other psychosocial care.

Scientists and scholars criticized Engel's model for one basic reason.[23] It advised only *what* clinicians need to know about the patient: their biological (physical disease), psychological, and social features. It did not specify the process—*how* to obtain this information from the patient in a consistent, efficient way.[24] Acquiring the necessary information seemed simple on the surface; just talk to the patient. However, communication teachers and researchers would find the solution to this process more complex—quite so, it turned out.

Before the biopsychosocial model prompted the idea of interviewing patients in a new way, doctors employed the *clinician-centered interview*. This practice of questioning had been customary since the start of modern clinical medicine in nineteenth-century Europe, when clinical pathological correlation was introduced. Doctors controlled the interaction from the start, often interrupting the patient's personal and emotional concerns with repeated questions about physical symptoms in a search for some physical disease. Most physicians still do this; you may have experienced it yourself. Perhaps you received no space to express your fears or interests, you may have felt depressed or upset that you couldn't afford a medication, or you might have had more questions to ask your hurried doctor.

The field soon recognized it needed a better interviewing model to obtain meaningful biopsychosocial information. Engel had himself perceptively addressed this in his 1969 textbook, *The Clinical Approach to the Patient*, as had early medical communication expert Barbara Korsch (1921–2017).[25] The small field of medical communication scholars at that time decided to undertake this daunting task: To raise the biopsychosocial model to the scientific level required, they would create an improved interviewing method that would procure the necessary biopsychosocial information.[26]

The Patient-Centered Interview Makes the Biopsychosocial Model Scientific

Influenced by person-centered concepts pioneered by Engel, Korsch, and Carl Rogers (1902–1987), the University of Western Ontario's Joseph H. Levenstein, Ian R. McWhinney (1926–2012), and their colleagues first created the *patient-centered interview* in 1980.[27] This method afforded the means to elicit the desired biopsychosocial information.[28]

Only gradually have many medical communication scholars painstakingly developed a scientific patient-centered interviewing method. Among the numerous advances, educators identified the many individual patient-centered skills and the interview's three functions: establishing a relationship, gathering information, and providing information.[29] Meanwhile, others developed a better understanding of the interview by the following approaches: working in basic communication research, studying the theoretical dimensions of clinical interviewing and a systems view, and evaluating the interview.[30]

Building on the groundwork of the many previous communication scholars, Ruth Hoppe and I articulated an overall model for the patient-centered interview in 1991.[31] I then refined and published it in a textbook in 1996, *The Patient's Story: Integrated Patient-Doctor Interviewing.*[32] The same year, Richard Frankel developed a similar method.[33] He and other colleagues later joined me to update the earlier textbook, now in its fourth edition and with a new, eponymous title, *Smith's Patient-Centered Interviewing: An Evidence-Based Method.*[34]

The updated patient-centered interview integrated many individual skills into a single, complete interview. Two randomized controlled trials and one recent controlled trial demonstrated that clinicians effectively learned the patient-centered interviewing methods.[35] In two other randomized controlled trials, it demonstrated an association with improved mental and physical health outcomes in seriously ill patients.[36]

In short, through a long, arduous process by many communication experts, the field had developed an evidence-based, patient-centered interview. The interview is considered evidence-based because it was successfully tested in randomized controlled trials.[37] (These research trials represent medicine's gold standard for acceptance as scientific.) Moving one step further, because this evidence-based, patient-centered method is what provides the content of the biopsychosocial model, this makes the model itself scientific.[38] In other words, the interview delivers the objective data that makes the dynamic biopsychosocial model scientific.[39]

USING PATIENT-CENTERED SKILLS

What does a patient-centered approach actually mean?[40] The term *patient-centered* may make it sound like a technique unique to medicine, but it simply employs basic interpersonal skills—the same ones key to anyone who wishes to effectively communicate and establish a good relationship with another person. Educators have simply adapted these basic skills to a medical context to facilitate students' and clinicians' learning. Any person can use these skills—not just medical professionals. You can call them person-centered.[41]

Try them with your spouse, parents, siblings, kids, friends, boss, or teacher—or even with someone you scarcely know. The results might surprise you. For example, after one of my residents used person-centered skills with his sister, he revealed his astonishment at her response: "That's the best conversation we've ever had; it seemed like you were really listening and cared about what I said." One of my medical students recounted a similar positive experience, though in a different scenario. He used them with a woman he wanted to date, and she finally agreed.

What person-centered skills could you practice yourself?[42] The key in communicating with another person, whether a patient or your spouse, is to listen attentively but not passively. While keeping your own ideas and opinions to yourself, pick up on personal comments the other person makes about themselves and issues important to them; what they say may not seem earth-shattering or even particularly interesting to you, but it's important to them, so avoid interrupting with your own story. If someone is worth speaking to, they're worth listening to, as well.

To draw out a person's ideas and concerns, you must show interest. To start, make eye contact and lean slightly forward to show your engagement. You might say something like, "Tell me more," or simply restate—or "echo"—what the person just said to focus the conversation on that topic; for example, "Your job's not interesting," or "Your classes are the worst," or "You're being forced to retire." These comments let the other person know that you're following what he or she said, that you're interested, and that you want him or her to continue on the same track. And remember, silence on your part helps. Give a person some space.

Identifying a person's emotion signals the peak of an interaction. Research from many investigators clearly shows the primary role of emotions is not only to maintain personal happiness and health but also to preserve human survival itself.[43] Accordingly, continue the conversation using similar comments, and listen with the intent of identifying possibly emotion-laden information. You can do this best by focusing the person on his or her comments that suggest an underlying emotion; for example, you might state, "Tell me more about your husband dying/losing your doctor/not receiving the promotion you expected/ failing a test/having your daughter ignore you/having three kids and a home job." Even if he or she mentions the topic and quickly shifts to another subject, return the focus to the possible emotion. Many will move quickly away from these topics; they are testing the water to see if you will respond to these clues about his or her important emotional issues.

Once you have reached the more tension-laden material and have probed further to better understand the scenario, ask the person about his or her accompanying emotion or feeling. For example, "How did that make you feel when your husband died?" or "What was your emotion when your doctor retired?" or "What was your emotional reaction when you weren't promoted?" Then draw out what feeling the person experienced to better understand it: "Tell me more about being depressed when he died/angry that your doctor didn't tell you she was leaving/upset about doing all the work and getting no recognition."

Sometimes the person will not initially express an emotion when you ask— he or she might reply along the lines of, "I don't know, nothing I guess, our family wasn't big on feelings"—but identifying emotions is essential. So try to delve further: for example, suggesting something like, "If that were me, I might be upset." When you say this, it must, of course, be genuine. When digging deeper in this way, use less-extreme words, like *upset*, *distressed*, or *distraught*, rather than more extreme-sounding terms, like *angry* or *depressed*. This is more likely to encourage the person to begin opening up about his or her emotional life.

Alternatively, if you prefer not to bring in your own personal feelings in your example, then you might refer to another person you know, perhaps commenting, "My father/brother/friend was pretty distressed when he had a check bounce and had to pay." Again, it must be an authentic statement, not an invention. If at this point you still have not succeeded in eliciting an emotion, you can remark—if true—that the person you are speaking with appears distraught. Once more, continue to use a less-extreme term for the person's distress: you might remark, "I can tell by the look on your face that you were upset." Interviewers using these efforts to elicit emotion usually succeed, so at this point, you have someone expressing an actual feeling. However, if the person still isn't, let it go. Don't push or make someone uncomfortable.

What do you do with the emotion you have witnessed? Make verbal statements of empathy. This maximizes your connection with the other person. Using the mnemonic NURS—for name, understand, respect, and support—will help you remember the following sample comments that fall into these four categories:

1. **N**ame the emotion.

   - "So that makes you feel upset/happy/angry/depressed/sad/afraid/relieved/ irritated."

2. **U**nderstand the emotion.

   - "I can understand that you feel that way."
   - "I understand how you feel."
   - "Anyone would be upset/sad/happy/irritated by this situation."

3. **R**espect the emotion.

   - Acknowledge plight.

     "You've been through a lot."
     "This has been hard on you."
     "You've got a lot on your plate."
     "That was a rough time for you."

   - Offer praise.

     "You have certainly worked hard on this."
     "That's courageous of you."
     "You're dealing well with this."
     "I'm impressed that you did the best you could."

4. **S**upport the emotion.

   - "Let's see what we can do, you and I working together."
   - "I am here to help in any way possible."
   - "You've got a good group working with you, and I know they've got your back."
   - "You have impressive support from your friends/pastor/team/family."

Everyone always says to be empathic or show empathy, but they don't say how; using NURS is the way. You might remember these empathic skills by adding an *E* to form the word *nurse*. The *E* stands for *empathy*, as nurses are famously empathetic.

Include the NURS statements repeatedly during the conversation, but avoid using all four categories at once—better to use just one or two at a time. For example, you might say first, "That's irritating [naming the emotion]. I get it [understanding the emotion]." After hearing the person's response for thirty seconds or so, you might then say, "That's been hard for you [respecting the emotion by acknowledging plight]." Then, after listening for another thirty seconds or so, you might remark, "I'm pleased you're able to talk about it [respecting the emotion by praising]," or "Can I help [supporting the emotion]?" Continuing to intersperse NURS comments throughout the entire conversation.

In most cases, the conversation should total three to five minutes. I'd avoid continuing it beyond ten to fifteen minutes, except in extenuating circumstances. After all, you're not a therapist, and you need to get your two cents' worth into the conversation to let them know what's on your mind.

I hear a common concern about engaging in these supportive conversations, so let me try to put it to rest. Let's imagine you have learned of someone's difficult situation: for example, a divorce, a lost job, or a serious illness. You may feel worried you've opened a can of worms, as you can't do anything to help. While perhaps true, hearing them out by being empathic ("NURSing them," as my residents and students call it) makes people feel better, whether you can help their basic problem or not. Many people in difficult, even irremediable situations make the point that someone listening to their story with empathy can offer the most relief. They don't want or expect that person to fix the issue. They just want to feel understood, respected, and supported. Identifying problems using person-centered skills and using NURS does not make you responsible for the solution. If you think it appropriate and feasible, go ahead and explore how you might help. If there's nothing you can do, then don't worry. That's not your responsibility.

Evidence Supports Patient-Centered Practices and the Biopsychosocial Model

An early review of many studies, including randomized controlled trials, demonstrated that patient-centered communication skills correlated with better patient health outcomes. These data also indicated improved bodily function and decreased symptoms, such as pain.[44] Another study by Western Ontario investigators found that improved communication corresponded with patients' perception of having established a common ground with their clinician.[45] Much corroboration would follow.

More recent studies of randomized controlled trials continue to demonstrate improved patient outcomes from patient-centered practices. For example, the rigorous study of numerous such trials concluded the effectiveness of patient-centered practices.[46] Other studies include a review of several randomized controlled trials demonstrating that a focus on the clinician-patient relationship was associated with many improved health outcomes.[47] A review of randomized controlled trials by Stanford researcher and psychiatrist David Spiegel even demonstrated improved survival in certain types of cancer patients receiving patient-centered attention, particularly when other treatment had failed.[48] In addition, literally volumes of rigorous experimental data indicate the effectiveness of integrating mental health care into medical care, using a clinical approach known as collaborative care, initiated and developed by University of Washington psychiatrist and researcher Wayne Katon (1950–2015).[49] Collaborative care has shown improved outcomes of such conditions as diabetes and hypertension when doctors also treat their mental disorder.[50]

Beyond physical health outcomes, studies from leading investigators show that patient-centered approaches yield improved patient satisfaction, which in turn improves patients' adherence to—or compliance with—treatment recommendations.[51] Other research demonstrates that patient satisfaction correlates with fewer malpractice suits.[52] Finally, patient-centered practices tend to foster improved patients' understanding and recall of their clinical situation.[53]

Some Medical Educators Embrace Psychosocial Factors

Many in medical education picked up on the initial advances of the 1970s and 1980s, with the support of the Association of American Medical Colleges, which prescribes the content taught at MD-granting medical schools. By 2001, the Institute of Medicine had identified patient-centered care as a key marker of quality, and virtually all medical schools and residencies now endorse the biopsychosocial model.[54] In parallel, nearly all medical schools now train their students in patient-centered interviewing practices. In addition, many schools now include training in medical ethics and social medicine.

The Association of American Medical Colleges has taken an additionally encouraging step: It now identifies which students will likely have a more humane perspective before they enter medical school. This is a major departure from earlier admission policies that selected students with interests and skills restricted to the sciences. To accomplish this new goal, they have expanded the requirements of premedical students' knowledge by adding a large portion of psychosocial material on its Medical College Admission Test, which undergraduate students must take when applying to medical school.[55]

Identifying more humane physicians marks a significant new direction. When taking these qualifying entrance exams many years ago, my fellow premedical students and I found no questions on psychology or the social sciences or ethics. We therefore focused exclusively on the basic sciences during our undergraduate education. Unfortunately, this strict concentration deprived us of the more comprehensive learning about humankind's humanity that comes from studying, for example, psychology, literature, theater, history, music, and the social sciences. Thankfully, the Association of American Medical Colleges today wants to develop broader-based doctors who value psychosocial principles.

Medical education has undergone similar advances in postgraduate or residency training. The Accreditation Council for Graduate Medical Education (ACGME) integrates the biopsychosocial model and patient-centered principles into the milestones and competencies it uses to decide whether residents are showing satisfactory progress during training and, eventually, whether they should graduate.[56] The ACGME has introduced respectful interactions, professionalism, communication, and doctor-patient relationship skills as part of all residency teaching and evaluation.

But a high hurdle remains. While these advances are encouraging, they do not include mental health instruction, where medical education has made no progress whatsoever, still no more than about 2 percent of total training time. Nor does the progress I've described here suggest great inroads. Most curricular successes involve patient-centered interviewing instruction in the first or second year of medical school—instruction consisting of no more than 2 percent of students' total curricular time. Then, in the last two clinical years of medical school, these institutions conduct minimal if any patient-centered teaching at all.[57] At the same time, residencies have added little if any new psychosocial teaching, other than a modicum in family medicine.[58]

Nevertheless, while medical education still has a long way to go, the biopsychosocial model shows significant evidence of challenging the disease-only model that has governed Western clinical medicine and medical education since the late 1800s.[59] The new model bespeaks meaningful traction with a significant base of medical educators, so a crucial foundation exists for future change.

The Paradigm Shift to the Biopsychosocial Model

What will it take for medicine to fully transition to the biopsychosocial model? I believe it will require strong directives from the public and its political representatives because, unhappily, modern medicine seems stuck. The characteristics of theoretical changes in other sciences corroborate this and can offer a sense of what factors drive a new direction.

Throughout history, converting from one guiding philosophy to another has been extraordinarily challenging in all scientific disciplines.[60] Even when long-existing theory repeatedly foundered, major scientific progress proceeded at a snail's pace. For example, discarding Ptolemy's (100–170 AD) earth-centric theory, advocated by the Bible, took nearly two centuries and the brilliant discoveries of Nicolaus Copernicus (1473–1543), Johannes Kepler (1571–1630), and finally Galileo Galilei (1564–1642).[61] Only then did science and the public accept that the earth revolved about the sun.[62]

If you believe that scientists are always logical and rational, then you're in for a shock. The first—perhaps surprising—barriers to major turnarounds in philosophy and scientific theory are an entrenched attitude and rigid thinking that lock scientists into their old mode of reasoning.[63] So even when research refutes a well-established model, the scientific establishment itself often balks—as you see now with medicine. Therefore, establishing that a new direction is the best way forward has always been slow. Demonstrating the existence of a better alternative means admitting the currently accepted ideas of some individual or group was wrong or didn't have the foresight to evolve. Max Planck (1858–1947), the famous physicist, captured the conundrum: "A new scientific truth does not triumph by convincing its opponents and making them see the light, but rather because its opponents eventually die and a new generation grows up that is familiar with it."[64] Put more succinctly, science advances one funeral at a time.

In the past, the second roadblock to adopting an improved model of thought was the lack of scientific personnel and infrastructure. However, this impediment no longer exists. Greater numbers of experts, better methods, and vastly improved modes of communication among modern scientists have extinguished the previous extended delays.[65] Because more scientists conduct research today, there exists a far greater variety and volume of scientific input for any given issue. Also, modern research methodology vastly outstrips early equipment; for example, compare the telescopes of Galileo to modern examples, like the Hubble space telescope and the new James Webb space telescope.

Finally, scientists' ability to communicate both among themselves and with the public is quicker than ever before.[66] In the sixteenth century, for example, scientific progress depended on the horse-drawn postal system. It could take six months for one scientist to learn the results of another and even longer for them to collaborate.[67] Therefore working collaboratively merely slowed progress. Only in the seventeenth century did any formal social organizations develop to facilitate communication among scientists; the Royal Society in London was the first, established in 1660.[68] Today, of course, these organizations are too numerous to count.

Now consider the impact of internet technology. Scientists can instantly communicate worldwide with multiple colleagues and conduct research remotely. And they can keep up to date in their now rapidly changing fields, often becoming aware of key modifications in their fields practically the moment they occur. Meanwhile, digital technology increasingly supplants printed textbooks, as online textbooks and medical journals keep scientists continually abreast of new developments.

As a result of these advances in technology and communications in the relatively brief interval since the 1970s, the public has conclusive evidence of the now well-known decline of American psychological health care and chronic disease care. Since then, multiple scholars have also identified the biopsychosocial model as a scientific way to lead medicine out of this trouble. Thus, in a short time, modern scientific investigations have already generated ample information to overthrow the Cartesian mind-body dichotomy. Even though the medical establishment seems oblivious, the public has the information it needs to demand a new way forward.

With sufficient information and resources today to support a new direction, I now describe what transpires in a changing of the guard in science. This will provide insight into the process of revamping medicine.

THOMAS KUHN ON PARADIGM CHANGE

The most influential thinker to study how sciences change their underlying theories was science philosopher and physicist Thomas Kuhn (1922–1996).[69] In 1962, he published *The Structure of Scientific Revolutions* and revolutionized how scholars think about radical advances in all scientific domains.[70] While incremental progress characteristically takes place over long periods within any scientific discipline, Kuhn noted that revolutionary, new scientific ideas occasionally emerge that can overthrow an existing philosophy and its conceptual framework. He called this process a "paradigm shift"—the adoption by a science of a new guiding theory and underlying philosophical orientation.

The conversion involves more than groundbreaking scientific facts. Kuhn maintains that, when the public feels dissatisfied, obtaining the people's input is crucial.[71] So what kind of events prompt the public and its scientists to adopt a new paradigm like the biopsychosocial model? Kuhn advises that only when the old system has descended into (1) abject crisis can such an essential transformation move forward.[72] He also says that, to replace an outdated theory, the public and its scientists need a well-established (2) powerful new scientific paradigm ready to take its place. He encourages, too, that the science in crisis review its own philosophical orientation, making its members fully aware of its shortcomings, and embrace a (3) new philosophical orientation.

Kuhn insists that science cannot continue to debate fundamental topics in terms of logic and research within the framework of the old theory. This makes supremely good sense because the new mode of thinking should sit outside existing knowledge and methods.[73] Unfortunately, modern medicine attempts to force-fit the old way of thinking into current circumstances by believing it can explain mental disorders via the disease-only concept: for example, the misleading belief that understanding genes and the brain will solve the mental health dilemma.[74]

Kuhn's additional criteria for change state that the new doctrine leads to a (4) possibility for new predictions not available in the old one. This means scientists will need to make significant modifications in scientific methods and guiding standards and establish (5) new guiding standards and methods; therefore, they must adjust their criteria for defining the legitimacy of problems and proposed solutions and determine (6) new criteria for definitions.[75]

Given these dynamic requirements for successfully converting from one paradigm to another, here's my analysis of our present status in terms of Kuhn's guidelines:

1. **An Abject Crisis:** There is no question of the current situation's serious state, including the massive numbers of unnecessary deaths, the severe disability in both psychological and chronic physical disorders, and the unnecessary spending of trillions of dollars.
2. **A Powerful New Scientific Paradigm:** The biopsychosocial model fulfills the requirement of a well-established, scientific model and superior replacement for the previous one.
3. **A New Philosophical Orientation:** Since the work of Engel and others beginning in the 1970s, a significant minority within medical school leadership now accepts the biopsychosocial model and patient-centered interactions.
4. **Possibility for New Predictions:** The biopsychosocial model imparts the capability for making many new predictions: for example, improved chronic disease care by treating a co-occurring mental illness and improving prevention and care by addressing such health issues as diet and lifestyle.
5. **New Guiding Standards and Methods:** Medical schools have begun to revise their guiding standards and methods in order to implement the biopsychosocial model and patient-centered interactions. Nevertheless, medicine will need a strong incentive from society to fully push forward these amendments.
6. **New Criteria for Definitions:** Medical schools have already exhibited some changes that meet Kuhn's criteria for defining disorders and solutions. But once again, the public will need to exact pressure on policy makers to achieve widespread medical recognition that not just biological but also psychological and social parameters define all illnesses and solutions in medicine.[76]

Considering Kuhn's six requirements, I believe imminent transformation is possible if politicians receive forceful public input. Reams of compelling research data already demonstrate the crucial first three conditions. The remaining three criteria will come to completion only with society's input. In my opinion, the public must actively engage at this point. In the final chapter, I present a specific political mechanism that can quickly operationalize society's demand for change.

Part III

WHAT PROGRESS WILL REQUIRE

CHAPTER 7

Impediments to Change

Progressing toward a new paradigm requires confronting three formidable hurdles: (1) a flaw in medicine's thinking, (2) the negative effects of individual and social stigma, and especially (3) the obstacles posed by the medical-industrial complex. The people and institutions connected to these three categories typically do not recognize their problematic actions, and this greatly increases resistance to change, making them unaware of their own choices on a conscious level; ultimately, they become unable to evaluate their options and act on a rational level.

A Flaw in Medical Establishment Thinking

The famous comment attributed to Albert Einstein (1879–1955), "We cannot solve problems by using the same kind of thinking we used when we created them," captures this stumbling block of reasoning perfectly.[1] It parallels the idea that medicine isn't so much unreasonable or stubborn as paralyzed by its disease-only mode of thinking when it comes to solving the psychological health care dilemma.[2]

What does this faulty thinking process look like? Communication theorist Paul Wátzlawick (1921–2007) and colleagues refer to it as "level confusion," the idea that medicine can resolve America's mental health troubles by applying solutions derived through disease-level analysis.[3] For example, medicine devised a number of ineffective means to address the vast population-wide psychiatric health care dilemma. Some examples: guarantee better insurance payments for psychological care by untrained clinicians, reduce competing demands on these physicians to give them more time for patients with mental illnesses, and provide patients with seldom-available psychiatric consultation with the doctor.[4] This type of flawed reasoning perhaps reminds you of the old story where an intoxicated man looks furtively for his car keys beneath a streetlight; when the man is asked where he misplaced them, he indicates it was somewhere in the dark alley behind him. Asked why he didn't simply look there instead, he indignantly replies, "This is where the light is."

Experts tell us that solving an unrelenting problem often involves altering one's customary process of thinking; many call it out-of-the-box thinking.[5] In medicine's case, this means thinking in psychosocial rather than disease terms. Initially, such a different approach may seem illogical or lacking in common sense because it will appear alien to medicine's familiar disease-level reasoning. Therefore, for medicine to make a major transition, facts about the new direction must demonstrate a path to improvement. And at the same time, physicians must experience the solution as congenial to medicine's scientific and rational way of thinking—as concrete and definable, not some utopian endpoint—with guidelines on how to achieve it.

According to psychiatrist Thomas Insel, former director of the National Institute of Mental Health, America's leader in psychiatric research, the field requires a different form of reasoning to advance and overcome a century of failure in mental health care.[6] Why? At present, the nation is no closer to a solution than it was a quarter century ago.[7] Contrast this to the dramatic improvements in heart disease care, where the rate of deaths has plummeted by 50 percent over the last fifty years, according to recently reported research in the prestigious *New England Journal of Medicine*.[8] Medicine's faulty thinking is especially apparent in its unidimensional focus on finding some explanation for mental disorders in actual brain disease.[9] Soberingly, Randolph Nesse, an evolutionary psychiatry expert, explains that the brain differs from other organs in being an information-processing unit; he suggests it is unlikely that researchers will ever find specific brain diseases causing most mental disorders.[10]

Problem-solving experts point out that practitioners and other medical-establishment decision-makers often exhibit another pitfall in their approach to solving the psychological health dilemma. They persist in addressing *why* it occurred rather than *how* to fix it.[11] To be sure, answering why can motivate you to seek action. But obsessing about why the problem came about will not point to a way forward, Wátzlawick and colleagues insist.[12] At times, this hazardous reasoning can lead experts to envision no solution—because why-oriented thinking inherently provides none. Sadly, many have lost hope of ever improving poor care because they erroneously infer that medicine and the public cannot modify their approach.

What, then, should a concerned populace ask? They must demand *how* to solve the predicament—right now.[13] I introduce a how-based solution to the mental health quandary in the final chapter and provide its operational details in appendixes B and C.

Stigma: A Bane to Patients, Clinicians, and Society

Society's negative emotional reactions and damaging attitudes toward patients with psychiatric disorders have created hurtful stigma. To help solve this predicament, people need to look inward and examine their own emotions. However, individuals often suppress stigmatizing attitudes from their conscious lives, unaware they are nonetheless acting on them—making the problem even more difficult to solve.[14] Stigma also has another dimension: the need to categorize.[15] While many find separating certain elements necessary to daily functioning (e.g., housing and eating expenses in one's household budget), categorizing people generates a concerning dichotomy of "self versus other."[16]

What kind of danger does stigma produce? People view the denigrated person with a psychological disorder as different from themselves. This skewed perception leads to discrimination, which in turn diminishes the stigmatized person's opportunities in many ways. Shame, victimization, and alienation increasingly dehumanize the unhappy person; others often brand them as inferior or even dangerous.[17] National Institute of Drug Abuse director Nora Volkow lamented the "chilling effect of stigma" on caring for substance-abuse patients.[18] Indeed, research from Kings College, London, shows that persons suffering discrimination often find it more harmful than the primary condition itself.[19]

According to the National Academies of Science, Engineering, and Medicine, parents subject children to less stigma than adults. However, one-third of parents still said they would not want their child to befriend a depressed child. Meanwhile, one-half of parents believed that treating depression would lead to discrimination and produce long-term negative effects on the child's future.[20] Such attitudes bespeak stigma. How can such attitudes continue in a society where up to one in five children ages three to seventeen have a mental, emotional, developmental, or behavioral disorder? Not to mention, one in three high school students report persistent sadness and hopelessness, with 19 percent seriously considering suicide.[21]

Stigma also works the other way around as self-inflicted. Depressed patients shame themselves and avoid care, believing they must simply act "strong and independent."[22] Furthermore, as many as one-fourth of patients expect depression to have an adverse effect on their friends, while two-thirds fear it will produce a negative effect on employment.[23] Patients with depression also avoid care because they believe their doctor simply isn't interested or will view them negatively—again, due to stigma.[24] The fact is, health care workers do display a high rate of stigma toward mental health patients.[25] Perhaps most surprising, nurses demonstrate stigmatized attitudes—even more than other clinicians do—toward patients with alcohol abuse.[26]

Members of the medical profession suffer from stigma, as well. Even with the profound stresses physicians have incurred with the coronavirus pandemic, few seek care for their increasing drug abuse and depression.[27] This "tough it out" attitude begins early: Depressed medical students—common in medical schools—believe other students will view them adversely; therefore, they cannot accept treatment.[28]

Pessimism prevails about the possibility of altering the underlying adverse attitudes that perpetuate stigma.[29] Though many have attempted to offset stigma in terms of mind-related disorders, improvement has been slow.[30] Not only do self-stigma and public attitudes need to change, but so do many of our laws, regulations, and policies reflecting it.[31] Such switches have taken place particularly slowly toward a variety of groups; just consider the arduous process the disabled, the sexually abused, or the LGBTQIA communities have endured to make their private and public lives moderately more acceptable.[32]

Is there anything individuals can do to improve this situation? Some evidence suggests the effectiveness of focusing on a person's unique attributes rather than that person's mental illness.[33] Journalist Dan Goleman and social neuroscientist John Cacioppo (1951–2018) advise that social and emotional intelligence—making oneself conscious of and responsible for one's actions—also afford keys to eliminating stigma.[34] These forms of intelligence develop awareness of one's shaming emotions around mental illness. Prominent leaders in promoting personal awareness, such as Hal Stone (1927–2020), Jon Kabat-Zinn, and Herbert Benson (1935–2022), find that mindfulness and other types of similar practices can help people observe that they stigmatize individuals with a mental disorder.[35] Once aware, an individual can decide consciously whether to act on this negative attitude—or make an effort to better understand the other person.

To answer why stigma is so omnipresent today, scholars look to Descartes and the beliefs of his era that still haunt many Americans, as well as the medical profession. The Scientific Revolution exiled the personal and emotional features of humanity, and this idea later spilled over into society at large, as Capra and Luisi point out.[36] Indeed, reason and rationality permeated the public during the eighteenth century, appropriately called the Age of Reason.[37] By the nineteenth century, the idea of objectivity reigned supreme, and much of the general population devalued subjective phenomena, such as emotional and other issues of the mind.[38] The idea of mental illness was incompatible with the core beliefs of the Age of Reason, and the public deemed patients with mental disorders unreasonable, irrational, and even "mad."[39] These patients did not comply with cultural norms, so the populace ostracized them.[40] As in medicine, the general culture dismissed psychological issues, leaving them to fester literally out of reach in society's subconscious.

The Medical-Industrial Complex

The medical-industrial complex poses the greatest stumbling block to accepting a new direction. Along with the medical profession itself, this complex encompasses hospitals, insurance companies, and the pharmaceutical and medical-equipment industries.[41] A common denominator throughout the complex is a "culture of medicine"—not fully recognized—that doggedly resists a turnaround. This culture underlies the complex's powerful adverse effect on mental health care.

THE CULTURE OF MEDICINE

While controlling and even curing acute physical diseases in the early to mid-twentieth century, medicine's practitioners and their professional organizations progressively developed an all-knowing, self-satisfied attitude that rendered the profession impervious to outside input. As exquisitely detailed by sociologist and Pulitzer Prize winner Paul Starr in *The Social Transformation of American Medicine*, a powerful culture evolved that permeates and dominates the medical-industrial complex to this day.[42] Understanding this culture is crucial to comprehending modern medicine, as recently well articulated by physician and writer Robert Pearl in *Uncaring: How the Culture of Medicine Kills Doctors and Patients.*[43]

How did this culture come about? The medical establishment took charge of how to define health and determine which patients needed care; unsurprisingly, the establishment selected those with a bodily disease and excluded those with psychological illness.[44] When medicine subsequently triumphed in conquering acute diseases in the mid-twentieth century, it was left to medicine—and the medical establishment alone—to decide how to furnish health care.[45] Doctors and their organizations came to possess a clear vision of how to conduct their practices—a vision that only reinforced itself, as successes continued in conquering physical diseases. Notably, external input never materialized. Medicine alone set health care standards and transmitted them to new students without consulting patients or others as to their needs. Because medicine independently evaluated its own achievements, physician-author Elisabeth Rosenthal insightfully called it an insular business that wouldn't police itself.[46]

I argue that this superior, autonomous attitude infiltrated the later medical-industrial complex players and that most fail to recognize the attitude they embrace or the harm it creates. How does medicine turn a blind eye to this situation? Despite the crises I've recounted (excessive deaths, poor mental and chronic-disease care, failure to prevent preventable disorders, and excessive cost), medicine continues unabashed and unabated in its narrow devotion to physical diseases. Confident it's doing a good job, the profession has convinced itself it needs no modification.[47] Furthermore, many propose it is too proud to acknowledge a deficiency and its vested interests are too deep.[48]

We thus have fallen into the trap that historian and political philosopher Hannah Arendt (1906–1975) warned the public to avoid: science driving policy without public input.[49] I would add "especially when it is vested in the status quo."

THE RISE OF MODERN HOSPITALS

Early-twentieth-century successes in saving lives led to the modern hospital movement—this, too, founded on a narrow focus on bodily disease.[50] The population initially regarded hospitals with disdain as dirty and fit only for the poor; in the 1800s, the wealthy received treatment at home or in spas instead. With medicine's successes, however, these institutions reversed course to become exemplars of effective, clean care for all.[51] Hospitals transformed into community pillars; they evolved into lucrative businesses that would grow exponentially, along with escalating successes in disease care. Demands for care rose dramatically over the following decades despite an increasingly impersonal and independent medical culture.[52]

By the 1960s and 1970s, medicine had emerged as big business in America. Prices for hospital services grew the quickest, increasing nearly 150 percent from 1997 to 2012, while physician rates rose by 55 percent. It's hard to believe that from $5 per day in the early twentieth century, daily hospital charges would average $2,607 by 2019.[53] While everyone knows that health care expenditures have exploded out of sight, few recognize where most of the cost resides. In 2014, the United States spent more than $3 trillion on health care; approximately 40 to 50 percent of this took place in hospitals.[54] Since the 1920s, a medical behemoth had evolved.

THE DEVELOPMENT OF FOR-PROFIT INSURANCE COMPANIES

The economic risk of health care costs became apparent in the 1930s and led to the first insurance companies: the Blue Cross programs.[55] The initially altruistic plans of Blue Cross were nonprofit and served everyone; their goal was simply to assist the public with increasing financial demands. Unfortunately, for-profit insurance companies soon spotted a lucrative market and eschewed the charitable mission of Blue Cross. They forced Blue Cross to adopt a for-profit status to survive, marking the unhappy death knell for beneficent insurance coverage.

The development of for-profit insurance companies cost the individual dearly. To maximize profitability, insurance companies no longer spent ninety-five cents per dollar of a person's premiums on actual health care, the practice of the original Blue Cross. Instead, that portion fell to 80 percent on average but sometimes as low as 65 percent.[56] This means the insurance companies devoted 20 to 35 percent of payers' premium dollars to administrative expenses. (In contrast, Medicare requires just 2 percent for administrative costs.) You've heard about high salaries and bonuses for insurance executives—the cash set aside for "administrative expenses" explains how they financed these.

With almost no external monitoring, prices soared as insurance covered physician and hospital charges. Insurance premiums rose, and compounding patient expenses, many companies insisted on large deductibles and numerous exclusions, particularly for preexisting conditions. Many patients found such charges impossible to pay. By 2014, medical bills had caused more than half of approximately one million national bankruptcies, more common than the business failures so frequently publicized in the media.[57] By June 2020, medical debt had become the largest source of debt in collection, averaging $429 for each US citizen.[58]

The unfriendly corporate veneer adopted by insurance companies and hospitals added to these institutions' poor image: for example, incomprehensible hospital billing with no relation to the actual costs.[59] How bad did this get? A researcher presented the details of one patient's emergency-room visit to the hospital's CEO and asked him to estimate the price his hospital charged. The CEO's guess: $5,000. The actual bill: $69,000.[60]

THE GROWTH OF PRICE-INSENSITIVE PHARMACEUTICAL AND MEDICAL-EQUIPMENT COMPANIES

Enter the pharmaceutical and medical-equipment houses—the last part of the medical-industrial complex influenced by a culture of medicine vested in the status quo. These jumped on the same bandwagon of insurance-supported, unfettered fees facilitated by permissive regulators and politicians.[61]

Prior to the 1990s, pharmaceutical companies manufactured inexpensive drugs. Their primary goal: to provide a social impact at modest costs. But the AIDS epidemic transformed this, leading to the modern price-insensitive pharmaceutical practices. The first AIDS drug, AZT, cost each patient more than $8,000 per year, a level significantly higher than any previous drugs for equally serious conditions. Other AIDS drugs followed that cured this scourge—but at astronomical prices permitted by the Food and Drug Administration (FDA).[62]

The FDA not only disregarded acceptable pricing, but it also relaxed its rules on the criteria for deeming a drug effective.[63] This meant companies no longer had to demonstrate an impact on patient outcomes. Instead, to claim a drug or medical device was effective, they had only to show some improvement in disease markers: for example, the blood sugar level rather than the actual outcome of the diabetic patient's health. Consequently, pharmaceutical houses obtained accelerated approval for bringing all types of drugs to the marketplace, deceptively rationalizing their high prices as necessary to recoup expenses for development and research.[64]

Physician and writer Elisabeth Rosenthal also pinpoints that the small number of medical-device makers—sometimes called "the cartel"—charges whatever they wish.[65] While Medicare paid less than $13,000 for a joint replacement in 2016, many hospitals charged more than $90,000—some as much as $135,000.[66] Similarly, some charge about $40,000 for a defibrillator, which consists of nothing more than a battery, two wires, and pads. Still more troubling, there is even less scrutiny of devices than drugs.[67]

GREED AND MORALS IN THE MEDICAL-INDUSTRIAL COMPLEX

Beyond the ethical and moral concerns in ignoring mental health care, a consensus persists among experts and the general population.[68] They believe that the medical-industrial complex has rigged the US health care system to favor its own lucrative interests over those of actual patients.[69] From this perspective, one understands why they want to maintain the status quo.

Modern medicine set its own disease-only standards and established the prices, so one cannot escape the haunting conclusion that its professional guidelines are suspect. One painful example justifies distrust. In the 1980s, the American Medical Association (AMA) *removed from its code of ethics* that doctors' fees "should be commensurate with the services rendered and the patient's ability to pay."[70] By dropping this clause protecting patients, the AMA, medicine's most influential representative, invited ethical questions of greed.

The US public should be gravely concerned when medicine charges excessive amounts for care. Doing so negates what should be a basic ethical bond between the medical profession and the community it serves.[71] Yet the new culture of medicine determines its own standards without considering the patient.[72] Nevertheless, despite the evidence, I—and maybe you—find it difficult to believe that the people and institutions devoted to health care are more motivated by profit than the care of their patients.[73] I find it particularly hard to fathom regarding individual physicians. The system perhaps, but not my doctor.

An Alternative Explanation to Greed?
Stanley Milgram's Research on Obedience

To evaluate whether greed is now the driving force behind medicine, I'll ask you to consider another subconscious influence promoting medicine's pernicious culture. I refer to obedience to authority, a concept raised by physician-author Robert Pearl and researched by Stanley Milgram (1933–1984), a famous American social psychologist.[74] Milgram demonstrated the extraordinary fact that ordinary, nonviolent research subjects readily inflicted excessive suffering on others when they follow a researcher's command.[75]

Milgram's research offers clues to how decent, humane people may follow directions beyond the research laboratory: for example, ignoring mental health care and costs regardless of the harmful consequences to those affected. Have you found it amazing the terrible things seemingly good people can do? For example, how do innocent soldiers go to war to kill enemies without remorse or oncologists administer chemotherapy to near-terminal cancer patients when there is no hope of benefit? The experiments of Milgram may explain this phenomenon, even though researchers do not universally accept his findings.[76]

Milgram's experiments in the early 1960s tested the lengths to which an unsuspecting subject would go in acting cruelly when following directions. His research assistants, dressed authoritatively in white lab coats, instructed unwitting research subjects to act as "teachers" and conduct a memory test on purported "learners" sitting behind a wall. The teachers could not see the learners, but they could hear them. Research assistants instructed the teachers to administer initially low-level electrical shocks to the learners if they hesitated to respond or gave an incorrect answer to a question on a memory test. Meanwhile, the research personnel had advised the teachers that a certain level of electrical shock was dangerous and another level was deadly. However, the teachers remained unaware of the setup: the learners were in fact actors who would receive no shocks at all.

As the research commenced, the assistants instructed the teachers to increase the electrical shock levels when learners answered incorrectly (these errors had in fact been previously planned). Most teachers did raise the shock levels—continuing as the learners cried out in feigned pain and unrelenting even as the electrical current registered in the dangerous and lethal zones on the gauges of a bogus machine.

Milgram concluded that demanding a person to obey elicits actions different from—and often alien to—his or her usual behavior when there is no outside expectation or command. If a person acts to comply with another's demand, then the perception of responsibility shifts—without the person even realizing this—to the individual or organization he or she obeys, such as a military commander, an employer, or the rules of the institutions of the medical-industrial complex.

A new viewpoint accompanies obedience and assuages a person's guilt. This modification justifies behavior an individual would previously have considered unacceptable; it rationalizes a course of action outside a person's usual moral code. Indeed, if it means fitting in, a person might be particularly cooperative, showing extreme willingness to obey and believe these actions were necessary—and, most disturbingly, that any damage to others was unavoidable, perhaps even deserved.[77]

A psychic peculiarity also accompanies this shift: an intense attention to the details of the task at hand. Concentrating on a competent performance prevents awareness of actions a person would normally deem abhorrent. Take, for example, the bombardier on a bomb run that will kill thousands; to avoid this reality, he focuses purely on the technical details of the bomb site and release mechanism. No longer distracted by moral unease, he will celebrate the victory of hitting the target, giving no thought to the lives destroyed.

But according to Milgram, all forms of morality are not lost.[78] Rather, the person's moral apprehension shifts to obediently living up to expectations; this often includes ascribing impersonal attributes to victims, signaling troubling lack of distress for other, human issues of concern. For instance, a person following commands might excuse their actions with condescending comments like, "They're just gooks/krauts/jailbirds/crazy people/hypochondriacs/welfare queens/drug users."[79] By stigmatizing and dehumanizing those they kill or abuse, people avoid confronting their own inhumanity. Sometimes they brace up this new, obedient morality by a sense of benevolence and value to the general public.[80] As the medical-industrial complex does, they believe they're doing a good job.

Milgram's ideas of obedience easily apply to medicine's dilemma regarding mental health. Within the medical profession, the physician, hospital, insurance company, and pharmaceutical/equipment house take direction primarily from the culture of the medical-industrial complex—not from patients.[81] An alternative explanation is that some members of the complex don't simply obey; rather, they identify psychologically and socially with this culture's narrow point of view.[82] In either case, automatic obedience to or identification with authorities perpetuate the medical-industrial complex's actions. That's simply how medicine works—adhering to the rules it has written. This creates a culture of conformity with no impetus for trying anything new. As in Milgram's studies on obedience, this culture makes individuals no longer responsible for their actions; they merely operate within the existing context. It's simply the way it's always been done.[83]

I've described this likely contentious explanation for what should be a moral dilemma for individual physicians and their medical-industrial complex leaders, not unlike individual soldiers obeying their commanding officers.[84] The truth of this idea, if any, does not justify the practices. Rather, it ups the ante for the *need for outside input to direct medicine back to a more humanistic orientation.* If medicine is this unaware of its submissive actions, then it desperately requires help.

CHAPTER 8

Society Must Step Up

Mainstream medicine continues to resist improving mental health care, unwittingly losing its very soul along the way. Meanwhile, the sad state of psychological health care only gets worse because medicine hasn't revised its mental health education in more than one hundred years. All told, the medical establishment carries on, spinning its wheels to little effect.

Deficient mental health care in America is a classical Gordian knot, a puzzle unsolvable on its own terms. However, Alexander the Great (356–323 BC) took bold, decisive action in cutting the Gordian knot with his sword. Like the historic warrior, the public and its policy makers now must take charge and usher medicine into the twenty-first century.[1]

Summary of the Problem: The Mind-Body Split

Between about 500 BC and 1500 AD, Hippocrates and then Galen led medicine in making the whole patient its primary focus, linking the bodily and mental dimensions. Unless you believe humans can lose all their humanity, then this greater-than-two-millennia legacy must live on deep in medicine's core.[2] During the sixteenth and seventeenth centuries' Scientific Revolution, however, the Catholic Church and Descartes led scientists in divorcing the mind from the physical body. The church would manage the mind, while scientists took charge of the body. In the late 1800s, clinical medicine in the United States adopted the mind-body duality, and massive treatment advances followed in controlling acute physical diseases. Over the next half-century, America would witness its pinnacle of medical achievement.

But success turned to failure as medicine continued to apply its measures for acute disease to America's newly predominant health issues: mental disorders and chronic physical diseases. Medicine ignored the crucial psychosocial issues that determine the outcome of these patients' health, resulting in the crisis that now wreaks havoc on American citizens and the US health care budget. Therefore, what began as dramatic triumph by the all-powerful medical-industrial complex has slowly descended into outright injustice toward patients in need of mental health care.[3] As William Shakespeare (1564–1616) admonished in *Measure for Measure*, "O, it is excellent To have a giant's strength; but it is tyrannous To use it like a giant."[4] Yet medicine appears oblivious, continuing to use its power in just this way. Perplexed readers may contemplate whether medicine has lost its sense of compassion, whether anyone cares. Has it lost its soul?

Medicine Needs Help

I'm afraid that, on its own, medicine is unlikely to adopt the new biopsychosocial model of medicine more meaningfully. Numerous requests to take this new direction have been ignored for many decades.[5] Nor will medicine otherwise modify its current attitude toward mental health in any significant way because the profession has too deeply integrated the largely subconscious mind-body dichotomy. For medicine to suddenly decide to solve the mind-body issue—and thereby settle America's mental health dilemma—a new logical perspective would have to emerge to replace its irrational, long-ingrained, disease-only view. The first step in a *rational solution is painfully obvious: train the doctors who provide the care.*

In fairness, medicine should be amenable to a logical approach. Indeed, most doctors proudly identify themselves as "problem solvers."[6] Logically, cutting to the core of the mental health situation would seem to appeal to everyone in medicine, even if it may seem difficult. Too demanding? Challenging dilemmas have never hindered this creative, successful, and erudite profession. After all, medicine solved the human genome, certainly a more daunting task than figuring out how to train clinicians to conduct psychological health care.

Yes, some may believe in medicine's capacity for logic and humanity. Nevertheless, *the field simply isn't sufficiently aware of its own adverse culture to function logically or humanely where mind issues are paramount.* The nation's mental and economic health cannot wait for the medical establishment to undertake these issues itself; multiple decades will continue to pass, as the system unnecessarily sacrifices thousands upon thousands of American lives and staggering expenditures every year. Aldous Huxley pithily reminded us, "Facts do not cease to exist because they are ignored."[7]

Society Must Take Responsibility

Why should you, the individual, and your elected representatives demand change? In my opinion, three reasons stand out, namely frustration and impatience with (1) faulty psychological and chronic-disease care, (2) excessive health care expenses, and (3) medicine's often-irritating, self-righteous attitude.[8] I believe the last of these reasons will tip the balance to fully activate the public: not taking your concerns seriously, having the chutzpah to contend all is well, and insisting that you be grateful for what you receive.

A frustrated, impatient, and dissatisfied populace—strengthened by social activists—can crystallize the will of its policy makers to lead medicine into the twenty-first century.[9] A paradigm shift—the final step of transformation—requires this kind of public involvement.[10] *Unsafe at Any Speed* by social activist Ralph Nader (1934–) and *Silent Spring* by writer, scientist, and ecologist Rachel Carson (1907–1964) tackle the topics of unsafe automobiles and environmental pollution, respectively. Both authors portrayed instances of major threats affecting the public, where the perpetrators of the problems resisted change; Nader and Carson showed that these situations improve only when public dissatisfaction forces leaders to act.[11]

Don Berwick, former Administrator of the Centers for Medicaid and Medicare Services (CMS), maintains that, first and foremost, the public will need to set expectations higher—*society can no longer accept the status quo.*[12] And raising the bar is possible. For example, elevated expectations produced such successes as the civil rights and women's suffrage movements.[13] This means the public and its politicians will need to make firm, explicit demands and follow them up with rigorous oversight to reverse the catastrophic state into which medicine has fallen.

In short, the public and its leaders must provide the oversight to make medicine responsible to the people's needs. Medicine will, of course, be a partner, but policy makers must now specify *what* medicine needs to accomplish; medicine can then decide *how* to achieve it. By acting decisively, society will facilitate not only improved care and financial savings but also the profession's rediscovery of what Berwick calls its "moral law within."[14] Only then can the former ethical relationship resume between medicine and the population it serves; meanwhile repairing this relationship will allow medicine to grow and mature as a profession—and reclaim its soul.[15]

You heard earlier how the general population itself fell prey to the concept of mind-body duality. But the public has observed the growing need for improvement over the last several decades. Today numerous public and private media sources inform the people of life-threatening, debilitating, and costly mental health conditions. The result has been to raise public consciousness to the daily ravages of poor mental health care, ranging from drug overdoses and mismanaged suicidal patients to jail and homeless populations afflicted with unaddressed psychiatric disorders. Closer to home, many experience lack of effective treatment by their personal physician—or inability to obtain care at all—and witness untreated conditions ruining friends' and families' lives.

As if the nation needed another reason to act, the American mental health system, already on life support, has now collapsed before the public's eyes from the strain of the coronavirus pandemic. With the COVID-19 pandemic's stressful demands, mental disorders tripled, while serious suicidal thoughts and alcohol use spiked.[16] Sadly, most Americans received no expert, professional help for the ensuing psychological tsunami.[17] Surgeon General Vivek Murthy of the United States captured the looming irony Americans face: "It would be a tragedy if we beat back one public health crisis only to allow another to grow in its place."[18] And more crises almost certainly will follow: Warnings emerge almost daily that greater challenges lie on the horizon from the ever-increasing likelihood of greater climate-change disasters, new pandemics, or nuclear accidents. All told, the public's need for skilled psychological health care will only increase as time goes on.

Given the COVID calamity's effects on mental health, the virus ought to end medicine's isolated interest in disease. Undoubtedly, if this pandemic has one silver lining, it has proven the mental health care system's failure to handle the national need—but only if this prompts politicians to act.

The Need for Federal Intervention

Over the last seventy-five years, federal interventions have surfaced as increasingly prominent in determining the big picture of health care; consider the resounding successes of Medicare, Medicaid, and the Affordable Care Act. Further, federal policies regularly affect current issues of national health care, such as drug prices, women's reproductive health, and immigrant health.[19] In a word, US citizens can expect the feds to play an influential role in health care going forward.

Americans can now hope this care includes mental health. In his 2022 State of the Union Address, President Joe Biden declared, "And let's get all Americans the mental health services they need, more people they can turn to for help, and full parity between physical and mental health care."[20] According to the prestigious National Academies of Science, Engineering, and Medicine, to achieve whole health and get rid of the disease-only model, "only the federal government has the authority and resources to oversee the changes required across sectors."[21]

Past federal achievements highlight the national government's tremendous capacity to resolve the mental health predicament. To truly sort out the current situation, the same courageous political leadership that led to the previous actions will need to stand up—buttressed by social activists and a vocal voting public insistent on better care. Simply put, this country has repeatedly demonstrated the federal capability to champion policy that terminates the mind-body split once and for all. For those concerned with the idea of federal intervention, science philosopher Paul Feyerabend (1924–1994) cuts to the core of my argument: "[Political interference] may be needed to overcome the chauvinism of science that resists alternatives to the status quo."[22]

A "New Flexner Report"

Our political leaders can find a solution in what I call a "New Flexner Report," the political strategy I've promised that can lead to rapid change. Politicians, inspired by an adamant public, would establish a *rigorous, multiyear review to determine how well present medical-education practices adhere to modern science standards.* The review could be conducted by a presidential commission; a congressional commission; or the National Academies of Science, Engineering, and Medicine. Alternatively, a private foundation that wanted to make an impact on health care could do this.

We have a precedent for this gameplan: the Flexner Report of 1910, which I introduced in chapter 5.[23] Led by Abraham Flexner, the Carnegie Foundation conducted a review of all medical school education in the United States. It found that many schools had not adopted the then most scientific approach to medicine, the mind-body split and its isolated focus on physical disease; instead, they continued to teach the old, prescientific ideas of the four humors and treatments, such as bloodletting and the application of leeches.[24] Illustrating the powerful impact of a nationwide evaluation of medical schools, the Flexner Report led to closing many prescientific schools and markedly raised the standards others needed to meet to train medical students in physical disease.[25]

It is time for a new Flexner Report. Just as the first one investigated medical schools' adherence to the standards of the Scientific Revolution, the mind-body split, the new Flexner Report would determine how well today's medical schools address the new paradigm of science, the systems view. You heard about its application in medicine as the biopsychosocial model in chapter 6. This new theoretical base for medicine, now well established for nearly fifty years, values the psychological and social dimensions of patients, as well as their diseases, thus appreciating and caring for the whole person.

After a rigorous evaluation of every US medical school for deviations from a biopsychosocial education of its students, the new Flexner Report would specify the changes each school needed to make to fully embrace the model. Given the present-day shortage of physicians, however, schools not meeting the new scientific standard would not be closed; rather, they would be positively reinforced to change via financial and other helpful incentives, as outlined in appendixes B and C. A new Flexner Report will provide the critical leverage needed to quickly redirect medicine. The payoff: alleviating the mental health and chronic disease crises, improving the financial health of America, and rescuing medicine's soul.

When society and its politicians can generate a new Flexner Report, then appendixes B and C present the more technical and specific guidelines federal policy makers and medical educators will need to ensure successful implementation of the biopsychosocial model. This will begin with the logical first step: train the clinicians who provide the care.

Societal Hope and Resolve

I want you to come away from *Has Medicine Lost Its Mind?* with two points: first, that you recognize the deplorable state of America's mental health system, and second, that you resolve that society's leaders and federal policy makers take action to correct this via a new Flexner Report. At the same time, I hope you can see a ray of light at the end of a long, dark tunnel: The simple expedient of rigorously evaluating current practices will provide the authority for beginning immediate change.

I also hope you will not see this book as a defection or diatribe against medicine or psychiatry. I belong to their ranks—and am proud of it. But these things must be said. Medicine needs help. Encouraged by forceful, clear-cut direction from society, medicine can mature and reclaim its now long-suppressed soul. This theme of maturation calls to mind the myth of Icarus, the story of the adolescent boy and his father, Daedalus, a brilliant architect, sculptor, and inventor.[26] Daedalus had displeased the king of Crete, and the king imprisoned father and son in his palace tower. Daedalus ingeniously constructed wings of feathers and wax to enable their escape. His intention: to fly from Crete to Sicily. Daedalus admonished his son not to fly too close to the sun lest the wax melt. But the overconfident, self-satisfied Icarus soared so high in his youthful exuberance that the sun melted the wax, as his father warned; the boy plummeted in flames to the ocean below, left to drown of his own hubris.

You can see a parallel between the story of Icarus and medicine. Renowned psychoanalyst Carl Jung (1875–1961) provides further insight. An essential developmental task for both a youth and young discipline such as modern medicine—a field that embarked in the United States just more than one hundred years ago—is to test their godlike reach. Yet society measures ultimate success by how well they balance this mission with reality and in turn develop from adolescence to maturity.[27] Medicine must mature and recognize the reality of the world it serves.

There is only one way to mature. When the public and its policy makers provide parentlike guidance and supervision, medicine will raise its subconscious attitudes to the surface, acknowledge the mental health problem, and jettison its damaging culture. Ancient biblical wisdom divulges what must transpire: "Physician, heal thyself."[28] By addressing its own mindset, medicine can reclaim Hippocrates's ancient bond between mind and body and heal the suffering of millions experiencing mind-based issues.

Appendix A

CHRONOLOGY OF SCIENTIFIC MEDICINE AND THE MIND-BODY SPLIT

Table A.1. Scientific Medicine Begins

Time Period	Clinicians and Researchers	Major Events	Mind-Body Status
5th century BC	Hippocrates (460–377 BC)	Birth of scientific medicine; divorced from the supernatural influence of Greek gods; imbalance of four humors replaced gods as cause of diseases; bloodletting used as treatment	United
2nd century AD	Galen (131–201 AD)	Scientific advances from Galen's prolific research and writings will guide medicine until the Scientific Revolution; strong influence of the Catholic Church; four-humors idea persisted for disease causation; bloodletting used as treatment	United
3rd–15th centuries AD	Guided by Galen's ideas for more than 1,000 years	Dark Ages of Medicine, governed by the church, with little scientific progress; four-humors idea dominated; bloodletting used as treatment	United

Table A.2. Scientific Revolution

Time Period	Philosophers, Researchers, and Clinicians	Major Events	Mind-Body Status
16th–mid-17th centuries AD	Andreas Vesalius (1514–1564), many later scientists	Birth of modern medical science with dissection of the human body; initiated mind-body split because the powerful Catholic Church insisted on excluding the brain; anatomists focused on the rest of the body; subsequent developments in physiology and chemistry followed suit; clinical medicine continued as prescientific; diagnoses based on four humors and bloodletting used as treatment	Separated in basic medical sciences, united in clinical medicine
Late 16th–early 18th centuries	René Descartes (1590–1650), Thomas Hobbes (1588–1679), John Locke (1632–1724)	Continuing to accommodate church doctrine; the philosophy of mind-body duality was firmly established and guided scientists to accept the mind as separate from the body; clinical medicine continued as prescientific; diagnoses based on four humors and bloodletting used as treatment	Separated in basic medical sciences, united in clinical medicine
18th–19th centuries AD	Giovanni Morgagni (1682–1771), François Bichat (1771–1802)	Birth of scientific clinical medicine from the human autopsy; identified organs and tissues as basis of disease and cause of symptoms; replaced imbalance of four humors as cause of symptoms and disease; origin of modern medicine's "clinical-pathological correlation" for clinical diagnoses in Europe in early 19th century; treatment, however, continued as prescientific, such as bloodletting	Separated in basic medical sciences, beginning to focus on the body and physical diseases for diagnoses in clinical medicine
19th century	Multiple clinicians	Developed and expanded the clinical-pathological correlation in diagnoses; exported to the United States in the late 19th century; treatment continued as prescientific	Separated in basic medical sciences, Increased focus on the body and physical diseases for diagnoses in clinical medicine

Late 19th century	Chemical industry	Developed first effective therapeutic agents for physical disorders, such as aspirin and opium; prescientific treatment measures remained prominent	Separated in basic medical sciences, further increased body focus for diagnoses in clinical medicine, beginning body focus in treatment
	Johns Hopkins University (1889)	First US institution to adopt European practices; focused on clinical-pathological correlation for scientific physical disease diagnoses	Separated in basic medical sciences, further increased body focus in clinical medicine for both diagnosis and treatment
20th century	Abraham Flexner (1866-1959)	Flexner Report of 1910 reviewed all US medical schools and led to adoption of Johns Hopkins's standards for medical education, with its isolated focus on the body and its diseases; schools teaching prescientific practices closed, while others made major changes to match Hopkins's standards	Completely separated in both basic medical sciences and clinical medicine
Early to mid-20th century	Researchers	Key discoveries, such as penicillin, sulfa, anesthesia, and surgical techniques, led to dramatic control and even curing of acute diseases; prescientific practices replaced in all clinical medicine	Completely separated in both basic medical sciences and clinical medicine
Mid- to late 20th century	Researchers in clinical medicine and epidemiology	Further advances in care of physical diseases, such as polio, AIDS, cancer, and heart disease, led to doubling of life expectancy by the end of the 20th century; mental illness, chronic disease, and other problems with prominent psychosocial features replaced acute diseases as major US health care problems	Completely separated in both basic medical sciences and clinical medicine

Table A.3. Systems View Revolution

Time Period	Researchers and Clinicians	Major Events	Mind-Body Status
Early and mid-20th century	Researchers for relativity and quantum theories, cybernetics, gestalt theory, and general systems theory	Birth of an improved scientific theory (a systems view) led to revolutionary discoveries in modern physics, mathematics, psychology, ecology, and biology; considered complex interactions of parts to form wholes, a holistic view all but medicine adopted	Sees mind and body as interacting and inseparable and a new way to guide medicine
Mid-20th century–present	George L. Engel (1913–1999), patient-centered communication scholars	Used patient-centered interview to define the systems-based biopsychosocial model as the theoretical alternative to mind-body dualism; reintegrated psychological and social issues to provide theoretical basis for including mental health and other psychosocial care as part of medicine's core responsibility	Completely separated in both basic medical sciences and clinical medicine, beginning reintegration of mind issues by some medical educators
21st century	Most medical schools	Adopted a patient-centered, biopsychosocial orientation but involved no more than 1–3 percent of total training time	Mostly separated, significant reintegration of the mind by many educators
21st century	Medical-industrial complex, clinical practitioners	Remained almost entirely focused on physical diseases; mental illness care and other psychosocial problems, such as chronic-disease care, continued to be inadequately addressed	Mostly separated, some penetration into practitioners of patient-centered skills

Appendix B
THE TRAIN-THE-TRAINER APPROACH

You know by now that medicine needs to train all medical school and residency graduates to be as competent with psychosocial issues as they are with disease problems. However, when medicine decides to implement this advice, it will not be possible because there are insufficient numbers of mental health teachers, by more than an order of magnitude. Therefore, in this appendix, I provide an overview of a way to achieve the needed numbers of teachers: *train enough primary care faculty to basic competence in mental health care so that they in turn can train all medical students and residents*—a so-called train-the-trainer approach. I provide the necessary details here for educators and policy makers, such as numbers of faculty needed, how much time they will require, cost, curricula, educational objectives and methods, details of faculty training and evaluation, and evaluating training outcomes. Additionally, I lay out the role of the planning group to oversee the entire program and ensure the eventual widespread implementation of a biopsychosocial revolution in medicine.

Educators seeking a more thorough understanding of teaching objectives and methods, curricula, and evaluation materials can find additional details in my previously published material, and they can find many other useful references from psychiatry, primary care, and geriatrics, as well.[1] But to start, two books provide the basics. The first, *Essentials of Psychiatry in Primary Care: Behavioral Health in the Medical Setting* (2019), describes the core curricular material that faculty, students, and residents will need to master in primary care mental health; the second, *Smith's Patient-Centered Interviewing: An Evidence-Based Method* (2018), outlines how to establish optimal communication with patients and form a strong patient-clinician relationship.[2]

The Train-the-Trainer Outreach Plan

The train-the-trainer outreach program comprises "outreach educators" and "faculty learners." The outreach educators are primary care mental health experts from across the United States. Their role is to train the faculty learners—coming mostly from primary care disciplines, such as family medicine, internal medicine, pediatrics, obstetrics, and gynecology—to teach mental health care at their medical schools (hence the name *train-the-trainer*). Once faculty learners complete intensive training, these newly expert faculty will train medical student and resident learners to achieve a level competence in basic mental health care. Problem solved.

THE TEACHING PROGRAM

The most common mental health conditions primary care physicians see today—depression, anxiety, and substance-use problems—make up the core program curriculum.[3] The goal of training medical students in mental illness is to prepare them as the *primary mental health providers* for these disorders.[4] Preparing students for this lead caretaker role in mental health parallels traditional educational practices training graduates as the primary providers for physical diseases, such as heart disease, hypertension, and diabetes. The new program will also teach students to make the appropriate referrals to mental health professionals when patients' mental illnesses exceed their expertise, just as practitioners do for patients with difficult physical conditions. To facilitate timely referral of patients to a mental health professional, learners will also receive training in recognizing (diagnosing) the uncommon, more severe psychiatric disorders, such as schizophrenia.

Good news awaits: An educational approach already exists, so educators do not need to develop curricula, teaching methods, and evaluation tools. This approach was developed through extensive research conducted by consultation-liaison psychiatry, geriatrics, palliative care, pain/addiction medicine, and primary care.[5] Because much of this rich research base targeted psychiatry and other specialist learners, our group at Michigan State adapted it for teaching clinicians. In randomized controlled trials, we observed significant learning through our educational approach, centered on what my research group labeled the "mental health care model." Additionally, we noted both patients' psychological and physical health outcomes improved under the treatment of newly trained primary care clinicians.[6] Finally, we demonstrated that, after primary care faculty were trained in mental health, they effectively trained residents in basic mental health skills.[7] This research led to the only evidence-based approach for training primary care clinicians in mental health care.[8]

More good news: Educators have repeatedly demonstrated that the train-the-trainer mechanism itself—now a universally recognized educational model—surpasses other means of outreach on a wide variety of topics.[9] Its key advantage: sustained outreach over time because the multiple teachers it trains by and large continue to teach indefinitely at the recipient institution.[10] Therefore, once policy makers and medical schools decide to move forward with increased psychosocial and mental health training, they have an evidence-based strategy ready to go.

How the Training Works: An Overview

Teaching involves two steps. At an average-size medical school, five outreach educators will first work together to educate forty-five new faculty learners in mental health care; this is because most faculty learners will have had minimal, if any, prior schooling, even in the basics of such care.[11] Next, the outreach educators will train these faculty learners to teach mental health care to their students and residents. Table B.1 summarizes the educational objectives and methods to guide the training of faculty learners and, later, their students and residents.[12]

HOW MANY FACULTY LEARNERS NEED
MENTAL HEALTH TRAINING?

Here's the immediate question: What is the initial number of faculty learners to train nationwide? Because Americans experience more psychological disorders than any other health condition—a crisis intensified by the COVID-19 pandemic—medical schools clearly need a major increase in trained faculty.[13] I conservatively project that, factoring in practicality and feasibility, mental health–trained faculty should—to begin—represent about 10 percent of all faculty. Eventually, I estimate that this number will rise closer to 25 percent. However, program leaders can only determine the exact figures required by reevaluating the situation once they implement the present plan.

From the numbers of existing faculty in various disciplines throughout US medical schools, I have determined how many new faculty schools will need to reach the 10 percent goal. The Association of American Medical Colleges states that 155 US medical schools granting MD degrees employed 189,846 full-time medical school faculty as of December 31, 2021.[14] These schools instruct medi-

Table B.1. Objectives and Methods to Guide Training

	Learning Objectives	Instructional Methods
	Following training, faculty learners (and their later students) will have the knowledge, attitudes, and skills to meet the following five objectives	
Objective 1: Communication and Clinician-Patient Relationship	Master the evidence-based, patient-centered interviewing method, including • developing efficiency • integrating disease-based interviewing • monitoring the clinician-patient relationship • diagnosing personality types • obtaining difficult information from the patient (sexual, drug, abuse, marital), working with a third person or an interpreter • Integrating the computer and note-taking • Solving difficult communication problems (hard of hearing, mute, blind, impaired cognition) and unique patient populations (geriatric, adolescent)	1. Lecture/assigned readings provided 2. Small groups: • Review interviewing method, practice with role-play/simulated patients, then use with real patients • Practice objectives in all health care venues (clinic, hospital) • Introduce personal awareness work as integral to these exercises
Objective 2: Basic Treatment Principles	Apply three models: 1. Providing routine information 2. Giving bad news 3. Shared decision-making to address negative lifestyle habits such as tobacco use, obesity, and excessive alcohol/drug use	1. Lecture/assigned readings provided 2. Small groups: • Practice conditions in the objective in role-play/simulated patients, then use with real patients • Continue personal-awareness work as integral to these exercises

Objective 3: Mental Health Care Treatment	Master the mental health care model for the primary management of patients with depression and suicidal ideation, anxiety, drug/alcohol abuse, stress and less-severe mental disorders, chronic pain and other medically unexplained symptoms, and chronic diseases with accompanying mental illnesses. Learn how this model can apply in the following areas: • Working with families • End-of-life issues • Cognitive-behavior and operant mechanisms • Psychopharmacology • Nonpharmacological interventions (e.g., counseling, exercise, relaxation) • Community resources • Cultural competence and health literacy • Referral to (and comanagement with) mental health professionals Learners will also have the skills to diagnose and refer psychotic, substance-abuse, and personality-disorder patients and to manage some patients with bipolar disorder	1. Lecture/assigned readings provided for all conditions in objectives 2. Small groups: • Practice conditions in the objectives in role-play/simulated patients, then use with real patients • Continue personal-awareness work as integral to these exercises 3. Special mental health clinical experiences: • Mental health clinic in medical setting • Inpatient consultation service • Inpatient psychiatry • Substance-abuse clinic • Geriatrics • Palliative care • Adolescent medicine
Objective 4: Personal Awareness	Develop personal awareness of previously unrecognized responses to the patient	1. Lecture/assigned readings provided: countertransference and emotion-laden material 2. Small groups facilitated by teachers and other learners in all venues, exploring the personal experience of the learner
Objective 5: Team/ Collaborative Care	Use patient and relationship-centered practices in using the chronic care model to work effectively with physicians, nurses, case managers, social workers, mental health professionals, and other relevant personnel as a team for improving quality of care and patient safety	1. Lecture/assigned readings provided: medical safety, relationship-centered care 2. Small groups • Discuss readings • Continue personal-awareness work 3. Special and routine clinical experiences in all care venues, in- and outpatient, and facilitated relationship-centered practices to promote teamwork

cal students and many residents (some residents receive training outside medical school settings). The following breakdown of teachers' disciplines reflects the almost-exclusive emphasis on physical diseases in their teaching:

- **Basic Sciences:** 19,730 faculty teaching such disciplines as anatomy, biochemistry, histology, microbiology, pathology, pharmacology, and physiology. These faculty teach preclinical student courses in the first two years of medical school.
- **Disease-Based Clinical Sciences:** 158,164 teachers specializing in anesthesiology, dermatology, emergency medicine, family practice, internal medicine, neurology, obstetrics and gynecology, ophthalmology, orthopedics, otolaryngology, pediatrics, physical medicine and rehabilitation, public health, radiology, and surgery. These faculty teach mostly in the last two clinically oriented years of medical school.
- **Psychiatry:** 11,952 mental health professionals comprised of psychiatrists, psychologists, social workers, and others.

Figure B.1 illustrates the lopsided distribution of faculty in psychiatry versus disease-based sciences. Among the entire medical school faculty, only 11,952

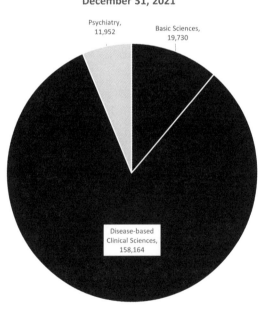

Figure B.1. US Medical School Faculty

Overview of Dissemination Plan

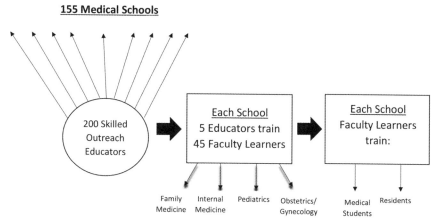

Figure B.2.   Dissemination Plan

members taught mental health issues. That's just 6.3 percent of all faculty and 7.6 percent of the clinical faculty who do most of the psychosocial teaching.[15]

To reach the initial 10 percent of mental health–trained faculty, outreach educators must prepare about 6,975 faculty learners nationwide. On average, this requires outreach educators to train 45 faculty learners at each of the 155 medical schools ($45 \times 155 = 6,975$). By adding the new faculty learners to the present 11,952 mental health professionals, the number of trained faculty would grow to 18,927—about 9.6 percent of the new faculty total and 11.5 percent of clinical faculty.

Figure B.2 presents the plan's overview. I estimate the program will need, on average, five outreach educators for each school and as many as 200 outreach educators overall. Though a major step for medical education in the right direction, this relatively small increase in faculty should allay any apprehensions that mental health education would overwhelm current practices.

INCREASING APPROPRIATE TEACHING TIME

While preparing faculty learners, medical school deans and their curriculum directors will need to decide on a required increase in teaching time to devote to mental health. A report from the Institute of Medicine gives clear guidance on the time requirement, reiterating the advice of many others since the 1970s: that medicine conduct *intensive* mental health care training in *all years* of medical school and residency.[16]

How much time educators will need remains undecided. Given that mental disorders top the list of common health conditions, one could argue that medical schools devote as much as one-half of total teaching time to the psychological and social components of medicine. Such a large portion is now out of the question because of the initial need to (1) carefully develop the framework for teaching mental health and (2) avoid political disputes that stem from asking for too great a change at the beginning. Therefore, to start, once outreach educators have prepared faculty learners, I propose dedicating about 10 to 15 percent of total teaching time to topics of mental health and other psychosocial issues—a major improvement to the present level of about 2 percent. As institutions continue to add more trained primary care faculty and mental health professionals—and the program's success promotes increased acceptance—mental health instruction can rise to 25 percent of total curricular time.

Where can medical schools find the time to add mental health to a curriculum already chock full of disease-oriented material? Once attitudes within schools accept a biopsychosocial and patient-centered focus, medical school deans and their planning faculty can, I am confident, resolve the logistics. Inevitably, many current disease-based disciplines will raise "turf battles" defending their allotted teaching slots. In my opinion, the best response is to convince them of the major advantages that can result from relinquishing just a small slice—perhaps 5 or 10 percent of their present allowance of teaching time. The fact that their most difficult physical-disease patients—those with co-occurring psychiatric illnesses—will benefit by addressing both disorders simultaneously should facilitate their agreement.

TRAINING FACULTY LEARNERS

I estimate from our experience that training will take about eighteen months, but this could range from fifteen to twenty-four months, depending on the rate of successful learning.[17] Based on our research, I further estimate that five outreach educators and forty-five faculty learners will require funding for at least 50 percent of their full-time salary, based on a forty-hour week. Both faculty learners and outreach educators will likely work twenty hours per week, but this should remain fluid to meet changing needs.

These twenty hours devoted to the program will break down into these activities:

1. Eight hours per week of direct contact between outreach educators and faculty learners: for example, a half-day two times per week or one full day once a week. During these periods, outreach educators will teach both on-

site and remotely; this might break down into several options. For example, they might conduct training on-site every fourth week and teach remotely the other three weeks of the month. Depending on how quickly the faculty learners master the material, this arrangement could vary, perhaps requiring more on-site teaching early on and less in-person as the program progresses.

2. An additional twelve hours per week for outreach educators and faculty learners to meet other teaching needs. For the former, this might include interfacing with the host institution to receive its input and gauge its level of satisfaction; they might also facilitate organizational issues, such as establishing a mental health clinic in all primary care settings. For faculty learners, this additional time might include preparatory reading, observing digital recordings, recording patient interactions for later supervision, and meeting with medical student learners.

EDUCATIONAL CONTENT AND METHODS

The newly trained faculty learners will supplement present efforts throughout all four years of student instruction. In students' preclinical years (years 1 and 2), faculty learners will participate in a much-expanded program teaching interviewing, physician-patient relationships, medical ethics, and social medicine, as well as introduce preparatory material for mental health and other psychosocial features of health care, such as motivating patients to adopt new lifestyle habits. Next, in students' clinical years (years 3 and 4), faculty learners will teach the core curriculum of depression, anxiety, and substance abuse during basic clinical rotations in family medicine, internal medicine, obstetrics/gynecology, pediatrics, and psychiatry. This will concentrate on patients suffering the following: chronic physical diseases, co-occurring medical and mental disorders, chronic pain and other medically unexplained symptoms, addictions, and post-traumatic stress disorders. It will also address the underserved, geriatrics, adolescent health, palliative care, and end-of-life care. The program will integrate instruction in both outpatient and hospital settings, including psychiatry, where there will be an emphasis of learning how to work in integrative health care settings.

In both clinical and preclinical settings, outreach educators and, later, faculty learners will use standard teaching methods, such as seminars and patient experiences. During *preclinical years*, these will include lectures and seminars on such topics as communication, ethics, social medicine, and mental health care diagnosis and treatment; preclinical training in communication and clinician patient relationships will feature both clinic- and hospital-supervised patient experiences. During *clinical years*, supervised mental health care experiences will take place in mental health clinics constructed within all primary care settings and in consultation-liaison services in hospitals.[18] This mode of teaching will be almost entirely based on direct experience with the patient and take place in family medicine, internal medicine, pediatrics, and obstetrics/gynecology in- and outpatient units. In addition, faculty learners and psychiatry staff will continue students' present instruction in both in- and outpatient psychiatry.

Delivering the Approach Nationally

We know that medical schools and their faculty will vary in their receptivity to the new teaching. After all, this outreach education means embracing something different, upsetting the apple cart of disease-only care they have taught their entire lives. Encouragingly, research provides solid guidance on how to disseminate and put into practice new ventures when some recipients show resistance and reluctance. Experts find many theories relevant to overcoming such opposition, but most believe Everett Rogers's diffusion-of-innovations theory the most useful and practical.[19]

First, some background on Rogers's work, which originated in agriculture. A federally sponsored outreach program in the 1940s developed multiple agricultural extension stations in Iowa that taught farmers to grow newly discovered hybrid seed corn.[20] Over the years a gradual, ultimately dramatic increase in corn production followed. Eventually, the Iowa outreach program played a central role in mitigating third-world famine.

But there's more to this example than a successful outreach model: It marked the birth of dissemination and implementation research. This research stemmed from observing the process by which different Iowa farmers adopted the new information—some quickly, others waiting as long as many years. The observations in the 1940s spawned extensive research into the ways institutions (and individuals) adopted new information in all walks of life, ranging from such advances as refrigerators, computers, and mobile phones to the latest fashions in clothing and new methods of teaching.[21]

Now widely accepted, Rogers's work showed the rate of adoption of any innovation to be a *predictable and universal social phenomenon following a bell-shaped distribution.*[22] His five phases of adoption, moving from fast to progressively slower rates, are (1) innovators, (2) early adopters, (3) early-majority adopters, (4) late-majority adopters, and (5) laggards.[23] The goal of dissemination and implementation efforts is to enter the "takeoff" area of the bell curve shown in figure B.3: around 15 to 20 percent adoption.[24] Once that point of adoption is reached, change becomes self-sustaining.

Here's why Rogers's uptake groups are so important. Each of the five has unique behavioral characteristics that predict how quickly it adopts an innova-

Bell Curve and Cumulative Curve for Diffusion of Innovations

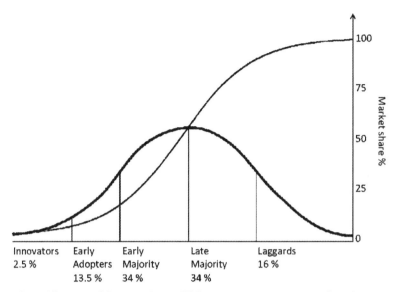

Figure B.3. Diffusion of Innovations. With successive groups of end users adopting the innovation (bell curve—dark black line), its uptake (cumulative distribution—light black line) will eventually reach the saturation level. *Adapted from E. M. Rogers,* **Diffusion of Innovations,** *5th ed. (New York: Free Press, 2003)*

tion. This informs which group one should—and should not—initially target for a new program. The first two groups are most important for launching a new effort; the other three fall into line later at the slower rates denoted by their names.

Research identifies the following unique features of the first group, *innovator organizations*: venturesome, open to doing things differently, receptive even to high-risk innovations, and ideal for feasibility studies. But as mavericks, they have less influence on wide dissemination. This is because they are usually small in size and at the periphery of their peer group, with limited influence on others.

However, the second group, *early-adopter organizations*, are established institutional leaders with prior leadership experiences. As such, they lend credibility to new ideas and communicate their successes, leading to uptake by others.[25] Research demonstrates that, while less venturesome than innovators, they possess such features as a receptive climate, openness to change, organizational slack that allows new approaches, and higher status. These organizations are often large and complex in structure but not highly bureaucratic, more influential among their peers, and highly attuned to what likely will benefit not only themselves but also their peer group.[26]

Here's how I recommend policy makers proceed. First, pinpoint innovator institutions to work out logistical bugs of the train-the-trainer method. Next, locate early-adopter organizations to deploy the program in its final form. The expectation is that these early adopters will then spread the word of their successes so that later-adopting institutions will be eager to apply the new model.

The Planning Group

From the outset, a planning group of experts in mental health, primary care, education, evaluation, internet technology, and diffusion of innovations will oversee all respects of the program. They will continue to do so until the program is adopted nationwide, transforming medical school education across America.[27]

For initial pilot testing, the planning group will first identify about twenty-five outreach educators—five to work together at each school—to train forty-five local faculty learners at each of five medical schools. Next, it will finalize objectives, the curriculum, and the teaching methods. The planning group then ensures that outreach educators understand the curriculum; particularly important, they must guarantee that these educators can teach the curriculum consistently and coordinate it with the local needs and interests of each school. The planning group will also organize and oversee the logistics of training both locally and from a distance in coordination with outreach educators.

The planning group will then arrange for testing the program at five promising innovator institutions. It will identify these institutions according to their readiness for change (per direct contacts), formal interviews, and screening surveys.[28] Throughout the pilot studies, the planning group will guarantee satisfactory progress. It will also make subsequent arrangements to distribute the program on a large scale to early-adopter medical schools the group selects and recruits; this will include identifying the necessary additional outreach educators. Finally, they will oversee the successful adoption and execution of the program at all remaining US medical schools.

The planning group will ensure quality and consistency of learning across all programs. They will develop a cadre of evaluation teams, and the group will also develop evaluation materials to quantify learning by faculty learners and, later, their students at each institution. Evaluation will focus on how well recipients learn the material, *not on patient outcomes*. As discussed earlier in this appendix, the plan already provides solid evidence from numerous sources of improved outcomes for patients.[29] Because research already has established the patient benefit, educators do not need to show again that the teaching improves patient outcomes in a new learner's hands. This is consistent with physical-disease teaching: Learners do not need to demonstrate improved patient outcomes after they learn about hypertension, heart disease, appendicitis, or delivering a baby. Instead, evaluation focuses on rigorous demonstration that the learner has correctly mastered the material.[30] Other experts agree: Neither the Institute of Medicine nor myriad other authorities recommended evaluating patient outcomes; instead they urged immediately moving ahead with increased training.[31] Perhaps they recognized the wisdom of philosopher Arne Naess, who emphasized the idea that doing something intuitively obvious—training the physicians who provide the care—should require no justification.[32]

Finally, the planning group will pinpoint additional activities for advancing the biopsychosocial model and mental health care on a national level. Such activities include how to train more psychiatrists, psychologists, nurse practitioners, and physician assistants; how to increase collaborative care and integrative care activities; and how to establish an agenda for rigorous research in biopsychosocial medicine that the National Institutes of Health and other federal and private agencies would fund. Given the current paltry and uncoordinated federal support for mental health training, the planning group will work to develop a National Institute of Health Education (NIHE); this organization would oversee consistent education in all respects, including how to best evaluate training.

The Long-Range Picture

My optimistic projections are that the pilot studies at five innovator institutions will take five years. Next, training at twenty-five early-adopter institutions will occur over the following five years. Finally, by the end of another ten years, the remaining 155 medical schools will have fully trained their graduates to a level of competence in mental health.

According to the Kaiser Family Foundation, an average of nearly 140 medical students graduate per year from each medical school.[33] At the *ten-year point*, thirty innovator and early-adopter medical schools will each be graduating an average of 140 fully trained students; this comes to some 4,200 (140 × 30) qualified physicians each year thereafter. At the *twenty-year point*, increased training will have spread to all 155 medical schools, producing 21,700 (140 × 155) competent graduates each year moving forward. Just consider that, over the next ten years, 217,000 physicians will have been trained. This represents a significant national impact because it finally places mental health and medical care on equal footing.

Sound like a long time? Policy makers have any number of additional options to cut this down. A more vigorous approach would enable completing the plan over a shorter period: for example, in five to ten years rather than twenty. And if policy makers wish to increase the plan's impact further, they could also train osteopathic physicians at thirty-seven DO-granting medical schools. Better still, they might also train nurse practitioners and physician assistants; their combined number of graduates per year slightly exceeds the combined numbers of MD and DO graduates: approximately 37,000 versus 33,000.[34] In sum, policy makers could reduce training time while doubling the plan's impact by training more clinicians.

But there's no quick fix, so look at it this way. Many have advised extensive instruction since at least the 1970s. Had medicine implemented the program then, the quality of psychiatric and medical care today would be on par with one another. A comment attributed to Mark Twain crystallizes the issue: "Twenty years from now you will be more disappointed by the things that you didn't do than by the ones you did do."[35]

EXPENSE SHOULD NOT STOP THE
PLAN FROM MOVING FORWARD

Costs will inevitably be the first objection to adopting the train-the-trainer method; however, this education will bring massive savings—from many billions to as much as trillions of dollars—to national health care spending. Nevertheless, it is undeniable that moving this strategy forward will cost money. My proposal for the initial pilot studies requires funding that is already scarce. Then subsequent widespread dissemination and implementation will require a much larger investment and a major reorientation of current funding strategies.[36]

Policy makers and funding agencies will likely find the train-the-trainer plan's savings of interest. Per our extensive database at Michigan State, the training of forty-five faculty learners at each of 155 medical institutions will cost about *$10 million apiece*.[37] The total cost comes to just over *$1.5 billion.* This is about $75 million per year over twenty years. By this time, when the later-adopting institutions have fully implemented mental health training of their medical faculty, all graduates will be skilled at integrating psychological and medical care. Discussed in chapter 3, this can save $28–42 billion the current health care system wastes *every year* by failing to treat mental disorders that co-occur with a chronic disease.[38] And these savings will pale before the far greater, almost-incalculable savings when these now-trained doctors address patients' psychosocially based lifestyle issues to prevent or treat chronic diseases.

Appendix C

GUIDELINES FOR SUCCESSFUL IMPLEMENTATION
OF THE BIOPSYCHOSOCIAL MODEL

What Leaders Must Guarantee:
Two Keys to Success

In implementing the train-the-trainer approach described in appendix B, policy makers must ensure that medicine also achieves two fundamental requirements: first, that it actively and meaningfully engages medical schools in the new program, and second, that medicine changes its present mindset. To ensure that institutions and their educators participate, they will require financial assistance. Happily, many schools have already shown strong psychosocial interests, promising that numerous medical schools will be keen to take part; nevertheless, these organizations must pay their bills. Policy makers will need to provide major financial support for schools' needs on a variety of levels. These include disseminating and implementing the program to all 155 MD-granting medical schools with multiyear financial incentives to both institutions and individual faculty for participation in and completion of the train-the-trainer plan. Further expenses include additional faculty time to conduct rigorous biopsychosocial research projects related to teaching; other academic opportunities attending the new outreach programs, particularly those publicizing the program's successes, such as presenting teaching results at conferences; writing books and/or articles for medical journals; and forming new administrative units to steer teaching and research efforts and planning the next phases in biopsychosocial medicine.

Next, policy makers need to be sure that the plan generates a new biopsychosocial mindset; mere expertise in the skills of biopsychosocial medicine will not ensure the program's success. To achieve this deep transformation, educational efforts must develop a *new narrative* that places psychosocial issues at the core of all medical care. This practice of identifying an alternative storyline to represent a new outlook addresses the most fundamental dimension of any successful change.[1] What will this process of conversion look like? As schools now deficient in psychosocial medicine evolve during training, they will assimilate the new narrative. Only this in turn can sow the seeds of a new mentality—an attitude that will instinctively hold biopsychosocial medicine as the schools' guiding principle. Indeed, as the new orientation clears out the old in medicine's subconscious, the humanistic, moral, and ethical changes sought by Engel, Berwick, and others will automatically take place.

Five Objective Criteria to Evaluate Medicine's Success in Moving to a New Paradigm

I propose the following five criteria for monitoring initial progress toward achieving transformation to the biopsychosocial model:

1. **Medicine begins a national outreach program to train medical faculty.** The profession begins this concrete action as a first step in a long-range plan toward implementing the biopsychosocial model. Consider it the centerpiece around which the following criteria coalesce and proceed in parallel. Parallel efforts will increase the number of psychiatrists and integrate psychologists into medicine.
2. **Medicine acknowledges its own role.** The medical establishment embraces its role, generating the confidence and motivation for a long transitional period ahead.[2] This includes stepping up and objecting to the present injustice of denying proper care to those with mental health and other psychosocial problems.[3]
3. **Medicine takes responsibility and assumes its duty.** The Association of American Medical Colleges, who govern medical student education, would most likely spearhead this step, along with the Accreditation Council for Graduate Medical Education, the body overseeing residency training.[4] These groups will operationalize the revolutionary new direction.
4. **Medicine updates its professional standards.** The medical establishment revises its professional standards to advocate safety of care, full access to care, and quality of care *for all its patients.*
5. **Medicine recognizes the social imperative.** Medicine reinstates the physician as a social instrument to address all the population's health care needs.[5]

Acknowledgments

I am especially indebted to the many patients from whom I've learned so much and who have stimulated me to write this book. Its intent is to crystallize a revolution in health care by inducing medicine to change to the systems view of life. Only this will provide significant respite to the difficult, now overlooked mental and chronic disease problems that ruin patients' lives.

I gratefully acknowledge my residents and their program directors in internal medicine (and some in family medicine) at Michigan State. The four hundred of them each had a one-month full-time rotation with me and my group during their first year of training and extensive contacts in their second and third years, as well. They embraced the new psychosocial teaching wholeheartedly and the research we conducted on it. We demonstrated its success in three randomized controlled trials and one quasi-experimental trial. My appreciation for their cooperation is exceeded only by how much I value the many friendships that developed. The teaching methods and research presented in this book could not have been done without them.

While like other American medical institutions that need to change, my training in medical school and internal medicine residency at the University of Iowa was exemplary and conducted almost without exception by caring, respectful teachers, many of whom became friends and mentors. Indeed, William B. Bean and James Clifton were key facilitators of my new direction when I left practice.

My practice partners from Des Moines, Iowa, taught me about primary care. Herman Smith, Charles Gutenkauf, Edward Hertko, Dan Glomset, Sam Zoeckler, and Jack Olds were the consummate clinicians as well as consultants. They also provided wonderful support and guidance for my decision to leave practice and pursue an academic career in psychosocial medicine.

Hal Stone of the Los Angeles Center for the Healing Arts played a crucial transitional role between practice and Rochester, especially being supportive and teaching me about relationships—and being a kind, caring friend.

There is much more in the book about the University of Rochester and Michigan State University, but I want to note some key people in my early development and success at each institution. There were many more than I list, but I'm especially grateful to the following:

Rochester: George Engel, Art Schmale, Bob Klein, Bob Ader, Tim Quill, Joe Messina, Leon Canapary, and Manuel Brontman

Michigan State: Ruth Hoppe, Pat Alguire, Scott Swisher, Ray Murray, Dave Greenbaum, Howard Brody, Bill Given, Barb Given, Gerry Osborn, Joseph Gardiner, Judi Lyles, and Rebecca Henry

Kathryn Rost of Florida State University was a key external consultant in many of my research projects, and she is the person who taught me how to write and conduct grants. I'm indebted to the National Institute of Mental Health, the Health Services and Research Administration, and the Fetzer Institute (Kalamazoo, Michigan) for large grants that led to the evidence-based work noted in this book.

Patient-centered interviewing plays a major part in this book, and I want to note several institutions who supported and spearheaded this crucial movement, particularly its teaching: Northwestern University's Program in Communication in Medicine, the Bayer Institute for Health Care Communication, and the Society of General Internal Medicine. Their efforts spawned professional organizations known today as the Academy for Communication in Healthcare, founded by Mack Lipkin Jr. and Samuel M. Putnam (1938–2005), and its sister organization in Europe, the International Association for Communication in Healthcare. These institutions led advances in communication teaching and research, and they spurred development of new waves of progress by increasing the numbers of those trained in the field.

Not least important by any means is my family. My father, Elmer M. Smith, was a general practitioner who provided my first medical experiences: for example, in his office seeing patients, taking care of me when I had nonparalytic polio, going on calls with him, and rushing to the hospital attending to survivors of a small airplane crash. My mother, Mary Louise Smith, inculcated into me the principles I live by, including the humanity that evolved in me that I note in the book. She also exemplified the critical, creative mind I so admire. Lynn Howell, my step-brother, provided crucial guidance and support as a key family member, along with my brother Jim and sister Margaret. My children, Becky

Beach, James M. Smith, and Julie Press, have always been my foremost supporters and have pitched in to read chapters and promote this book on my website.

My wife, Susan Sleeper-Smith, is the most remarkable woman. She's a skilled Native American historian with multiple books and papers, yet she has put me and my book first. She read and carefully critiqued my drafts with consummate expertise. On a broader note, she's what makes my life worth living in so many other ways.

In the actual writing of the book, I've had great advice on how to develop it from Alice Dreger, Lisa Tener, Janie Harper, and Mark Malatesta. The following readers helped tremendously in critiquing the book: Dave Sluyter, Steve Frankel, Howard Brody, James Smith, Judi Lyles, Ron Rosenberg, Josh Cole, Tim Quill, Rich Frankel, Brenda Lepisto, Mark Sullivan, and Susan Bandes. I also had considerable help from the Michigan State IT people, especially Allison Virag-McCann and Amin Elrashid. And my website could never have been developed without the diligent work of Dean Rehberger, Michaela Kaliniak, and Kayla VanDyke—and, later, Austin Sager.

I cannot say enough about my intrepid agent, Regina Ryan, in guiding revisions, with the skillful assistance of Abigail Wilentz, and in supporting me through a daunting, unfamiliar process. Jonathan Kurtz of Prometheus Books then took the book under his experienced wing. With the help of production editor Nicole Carty and copyeditor Niki Guinan, the book rolled out in a timely fashion. And my publicist, Joanne McCall, expertly guided the dissemination process from there.

Notes

Chapter 1

1. National Alliance on Mental Illness, *Prevalences of Illnesses: Support, Advocacy, Education, Research* (Gainesville, FL: National Alliance on Mental Illness, 2014).

2. R. C. Kessler, P. Berglund, O. Demler, R. Jin, K. R. Merikangas, and E. E. Walters, "Lifetime Prevalence and Age-of-Onset Distributions of DSM-IV Disorders in the National Comorbidity Survey Replication," *Archives of General Psychiatry* 62, no. 6 (June 2005): 593–602, https://doi.org/10.1001/archpsyc.62.6.593; G. S. Norquist and D. A. Regier, "The Epidemiology of Psychiatric Disorders and the De Facto Mental Health Care System," *Annual Review of Medicine* 47 (1996): 473–79, https://doi.org/10.1146/annurev.med.47.1.473.

3. R. C. Kessler, W. T. Chiu, O. Demler, and E. E. Walters, "Prevalence, Severity, and Comorbidity of 12-Month DSM-IV Disorders in the National Comorbidity Survey Replication," *Archives of General Psychiatry* 62, no. 6 (June 2005): 617–27, https://doi.org/10.1001/archpsyc.62.6.617.

4. National Alliance on Mental Illness, "Mental Health by the Numbers," updated April 2023, https://www.nami.org/mhstats; Substance Abuse and Mental Health Services Administration, "2019–2020 National Survey on Drug Use and Health: Model-Based Prevalence Estimates (50 States and the District of Columbia)," December 29, 2021, https://www.samhsa.gov/data/report/2019-2020-nsduh-state-prevalence-estimates.

5. N. Counts, "Behavioral Health Care in the United States: How It Works and Where It Falls Short," Commonwealth Fund, September 7, 2022, https://doi.org/10.26099/txpy-va3.

6. Department of Health and Human Services, *Healthy People 2020* (Washington, DC: Department of Health and Human Services, 2017); Department of Health and Human Services, *Mental Health and Mental Disorders: Healthy People 2010* (Washington, DC: US Government Printing Office, 2000).

7. R. C. Kessler, O. Demler, R. G. Frank, M. Olfson, H. A. Pincus, E. E. Walters, P. Wang, K. B. Wells, and A. M. Zaslavsky, "Prevalence and Treatment of Mental Dis-

orders, 1990 to 2003," *New England Journal of Medicine* 352, no. 24 (June 16, 2005): 2515–23; https://doi.org/10.1056/NEJMsa043266.

8. Department of Health and Human Services, *Healthy People 2010: Understanding and Improving Health*, 2nd ed. (Washington, DC: US Government Printing Office, 2000); Department of Health and Human Services, *Mental Health and Mental Disorders*.

9. R. J. Baldessarini, L. Tondo, M. Pinna, N. Nuñez, and G. H. Vázquez, "Suicidal Risk Factors in Major Affective Disorders," *British Journal of Psychiatry* 215, no. 4 (2019): 621–26, https://doi.org/10.1192/bjp.2019.167.

10. Baldessarini et al., "Suicidal Risk Factors"; W. M. Compton, Y. F. Thomas, F. S. Stinson, and B. F. Grant, "Prevalence, Correlates, Disability, and Comorbidity of DSM-IV Drug Abuse and Dependence in the United States: Results from the National Epidemiologic Survey on Alcohol and Related Conditions," *Archives of General Psychiatry* 64, no. 5 (May 2007): 566–76, https://doi.org/10.1001/archpsyc.64.5.566; L. Fisher and D. C. Ransom, "Developing a Strategy for Managing Behavioral Health Care within the Context of Primary Care," *Archives of Family Medicine* 6, no. 4 (July–August 1997): 324–33, https://doi.org/10.1001/archfami.6.4.324.

11. C. M. Smith, "Origin and Uses of Primum Non Nocere—Above All, Do No Harm!" *Journal of Clinical Pharmacology* 45, no. 4 (April 2005): 371–77, https://doi .org/10.1177/0091270004273680.

12. *Merriam-Webster Dictionary*, "Vade mecum," accessed June 6, 2024, https:// www.merriam-webster.com/dictionary/vade%20mecum.

13. G. L. Engel, "The Need for a New Medical Model: A Challenge for Biomedicine," *Science* 196, no. 4286 (April 8, 1977): 129–36, https://doi.org/10.1126/science.847460.

14. R. C. Smith, J. C. Gardiner, Z. Luo, S. Schooley, L. Lamerato, and K. Rost, "Primary Care Physicians Treat Somatization," *Journal of General Internal Medicine* 24, no. 7 (July 2009): 829–32, https://doi.org/10.1007/s11606-009-0992-y; R. C. Smith and R. B. Hoppe, "The Patient's Story: Integrating the Patient- and Physician-Centered Approaches to Interviewing," *Annals of Internal Medicine* 115, no. 6 (1991): 470–77, https://doi.org/10.7326/0003-4819-115-6-470; R. C. Smith, H. Laird-Fick, F. C. Dwamena, L. Freilich, B. Mavis, K. Grayson-Sneed, D. D'Mello, M. Spoolstra, and D. Solomon, "Teaching Residents Mental Health Care," *Patient Education and Counseling* 101, no. 12 (December 2018): 2145–55, https://doi.org/10.1016/j.pec.2018.07.023; R. C. Smith, J. S. Lyles, J. C. Gardiner, C. Sirbu, A. Hodges, C. Collins, F. C. Dwamena et al., "Primary Care Clinicians Treat Patients with Medically Unexplained Symptoms: A Randomized Controlled Trial," *Journal of General Internal Medicine* 21, no. 7 (July 2006): 671–77, https://doi.org/10.1111/j.1525-1497.2006.00460.x; R. C. Smith, J. S. Lyles, J. Mettler, B. E. Stoffelmayr, L. F. Van Egeren, A. A. Marshall, J. C. Gardiner et al., "The Effectiveness of Intensive Training for Residents in Interviewing: A Randomized, Controlled Study," *Annals of Internal Medicine* 128, no. 2 (January 15, 1998): 118–26, https://doi.org/10.7326/0003-4819-128-2-199801150-00008.

15. A. H. Fortin VI, F. C. Dwamena, R. M. Frankel, B. L. Lepisto, and R. C. Smith, *Smith's Patient-Centered Interviewing: An Evidence-Based Method*, 4th ed. (New York: McGraw-Hill Education, 2018).

16. R. C. Smith, D. D'Mello, G. G. Osborn, L. Freilich, F. C. Dwamena, and H. Laird-Fick, *Essentials of Psychiatry in Primary Care: Behavioral Health in the Medical Setting* (New York: McGraw Hill Education, 2019).

Chapter 2

1. American Public Health Association, "Congress Approves $1.1 Billion in Funding to Combat Zika," 2016.

2. Center for Disease Control and Prevention, "Coronavirus Disease, Coping with Stress," 2020.

3. Committee on the Science of Changing Behavioral Health Social Norms, *Ending Discrimination against People with Mental and Substance Use Disorders: The Evidence for Stigma Change* (Washington, DC: National Academies Press, 2016).

4. T. F. Bishop, J. K. Seirup, H. A. Pincus, and J. S. Ross, "Population of US Practicing Psychiatrists Declined, 2003–13, Which May Help Explain Poor Access to Mental Health Care," *Health Affairs* 35, no. 7 (July 2016): 1271–77, https://doi.org/10.1377/hlthaff.2015.1643; N. Panchal, H. Saunders, R. Rudowitz, and C. Cox, "The Implications of COVID-19 for Mental Health and Substance Use," Kaiser Family Foundation, March 20, 2023, https://www.kff.org/coronavirus-covid-19/issue-brief/the-implications-of-covid-19-for-mental-health-and-substance-use/.

5. Bureau of Health Workforce, "Behavioral Health Workforce Projections, 2017–2030," Health Resources and Services Administration, accessed June 7, 2024, https://bhw.hrsa.gov/sites/default/files/bureau-health-workforce/data-research/bh-workforce-projections-fact-sheet.pdf.

6. P. S. Wang, M. Lane, M. Olfson, H. A. Pincus, K. B. Wells, and R. C. Kessler, "Twelve-Month Use of Mental Health Services in the United States: Results from the National Comorbidity Survey Replication," *Archives of General Psychiatry* 62, no. 6 (June 2005): 629–40, https://doi.org/10.1001/archpsyc.62.6.629.

7. R. A. Crowley, N. Kirschner, and Health and Public Policy Committee of the American College of Physicians, "The Integration of Care for Mental Health, Substance Abuse, and Other Behavioral Health Conditions into Primary Care: Executive Summary of an American College of Physicians Position Paper," *Annals of Internal Medicine* 163, no. 4 (August 18, 2015): 298–99, https://doi.org/10.7326/M15-0510.

8. T. R. Insel, "Psychiatry: Where Are We Going?" *Director's Blog* (blog), June 3, 2011.

9. Bureau of Health Workforce, "Behavioral Health Workforce Projections"; A. Satiani, J. Niedermier, B. Satiani, and D. P. Svendsen, "Projected Workforce of Psychiatrists in the United States: A Population Analysis," *Psychiatric Services* 69, no. 6 (June 1, 2018): 710–13, https://doi.org/10.1176/appi.ps.201700344.

10. B. J. Burns, J. E. Scott, J. D. Burke Jr., and L. G. Kessler, "Mental Health Training of Primary Care Residents: A Review of Recent Literature (1974–1981)," *General Hospital Psychiatry* 5, no. 3 (September 1983): 157–69, https://doi.org/10.1016/0163-8343(83)90051-8.

11. Bishop et al., "Population of US Practicing Psychiatrists."

12. P. J. Cunningham, "Beyond Parity: Primary Care Physicians' Perspectives on Access to Mental Health Care," *Health Affairs* 28, no. 3 (May–June 2009): w490–501, https://doi.org/10.1377/hlthaff.28.3.w490.

13. J. P. Morrisey, K. C. Thomas, A. R. Ellis, and T. R. Konrad, *Development of a New Method for Designation of Mental Health Professional Shortage Areas* (Chapel Hill: Cecil G. Sheps Center for Health Services Research, University of North Carolina at Chapel Hill, December 21, 2007), https://www.shepscenter.unc.edu/wp-content/up loads/2013/12/Development-of-a-New-Methodology-for-Mental-Health-Professional -Shortage-Designation.pdf.

14. A. Mauri, M. Gaiser, J. Buche, and A. J. Beck, *Behavioral Health Provider Geographic Distribution and Reimbursement Inequities* (Ann Arbor: School of Public Health Behavioral Health Workforce Research Center, December 2019), https://www.behav ioralhealthworkforce.org/wp-content/uploads/2019/12/Y4-P9-BHWRC-Distribution -and-Reimbursement-Inequities-Full-Report.pdf; J. M. Richards and G. D. Gottfredson, "Geographic Distribution of US Psychologists: A Human Ecological Analysis," *American Psychologist* 33, no. 1 (1978): 1–9, https://doi.org/10.1037/0003-066X.33.1.1.

15. Bishop et al., "Population of US Practicing Psychiatrists"; Insel, "Psychiatry."

16. R. C. Kessler, P. Berglund, O. Demler, R. Jin, K. R. Merikangas, and E. E. Walters, "Lifetime Prevalence and Age-of-Onset Distributions of DSM-IV Disorders in the National Comorbidity Survey Replication," *Archives of General Psychiatry* 62, no. 6 (June 2005): 593–602, https://doi.org/10.1001/archpsyc.62.6.593; R. C. Kessler, O. Demler, R. G. Frank, M. Olfson, H. A. Pincus, E. E. Walters, P. Wang, K. B. Wells, and A. M. Zaslavsky, "Prevalence and Treatment of Mental Disorders, 1990 to 2003," *New England Journal of Medicine* 352, no. 24 (June 16, 2005): 2515–23, https://doi .org/10.1056/NEJMsa043266; G. S. Norquist and D. A. Regier, "The Epidemiology of Psychiatric Disorders and the De Facto Mental Health Care System," *Annual Review of Medicine* 47 (February 1996): 473–79, https://doi.org/10.1146/annurev.med.47.1.473.

17. H. L. McQuistion and R. Zinns, "Workloads in Clinical Psychiatry: Another Way," *Psychiatric Services* 70, no. 10 (October 1, 2019): 963–66, https://doi.org/10 .1176/appi.ps.201900125.

18. M. J. Goldacre, S. Fazel, F. Smith, and T. Lambert, "Choice and Rejection of Psychiatry as a Career: Surveys of UK Medical Graduates from 1974 to 2009," *British Journal of Psychiatry* 202, no. 3 (March 2013): 228–34, https://doi.org/10.1192/bjp .bp.112.111153.

19. J. Crabb, L. Barber, and N. Masson, "Shrink Rethink: Rebranding Psychiatry," *British Journal of Psychiatry* 211, no. 5 (November 2017): 259–61, https://doi.org/10 .1192/bjp.bp.116.197210.

20. Crowley, Kirschner, and Health and Public Policy Committee of the American College of Physicians, "Integration of Care."

21. R. Pearl, *Uncaring: How the Culture of Medicine Kills Doctors and Patients* (New York: PublicAffairs, 2021); P. Starr, *The Social Transformation of American Medicine* (New York: Basic Books, 1982); M. Sullivan, *The Patient as Agent of Health and Health Care* (New York: Oxford University Press, 2017).

22. Bureau of Health Workforce, "Behavioral Health Workforce Projections"; Wang et al., "Twelve-Month Use."

23. J. Caccavale, J. L. Reeves, and J. Wiggins, *The Impact of Psychiatric Shortage on Patient Care and Mental Health Policy: The Silent Shortage That Can No Longer Be Ignored* (n.p.: American Board of Behavioral Healthcare Practice, 2012).

24. E. L. Ross, S. Vijan, E. M. Miller, M. Valenstein, K. Zivin, "The Cost-Effectiveness of Cognitive Behavioral Therapy versus Second-Generation Antidepressants for Initial Treatment of Major Depressive Disorder in the United States: A Decision Analytic Model," *Annals of Internal Medicine* 171, no. 11 (December 3, 2019): 785–95, https://doi.org/10.7326/m18-1480.

25. American Psychological Association, "About Prescribing Psychologists," updated January 2022, https://www.apaservices.org/practice/advocacy/authority/prescribing-psychologists; Psychologist Licensing Amendments, H.B. 289, State of Utah (February 10, 2011), https://le.utah.gov/~2011/bills/hbillint/hb0289.htm.

26. Consortium for Advanced Psychology Training (CAPT), "Postdoctoral Psychology," 2018; S. H. McDaniel, C. L. Grus, B. A. Cubic, C. L. Hunter, L. K. Kearney, C. C. Schuman, M. J. Karel et al., "Competencies for Psychology Practice in Primary Care," *American Psychologist* 69, no. 4 (May–June 2014): 409–29, https://doi.org/10.1037/a0036072.

27. CAPT, "Postdoctoral Psychology."

28. R. Kathol, S. Melek, S. Sargent, L. Sacks, and K. K. Patel, "Non-Traditional Mental Health and Substance Use Disorder Services as a Core Part of Health in CINs and ACOs," in *Clinical Integration: Population Health and Accountable Care*, 3rd ed., ed. K. Yale, T. A. Raskauskas, J. Bohn, and C. Konschak, 380–425 (Virginia Beach, VA: Convergent 2015); S. Melek and D. Norris, *Chronic Conditions and Comorbid Psychological Disorders*, Milliman Research Report (Seattle, WA: Milliman, July 2008), https://www.cbhc.org/wp-content/uploads/2015/11/chronic-conditions-and-comorbid-RR07-01-08.pdf; P. S. Wang, O. Demler, M. Olfson, H. A. Pincus, K. B. Wells, and R. C. Kessler, "Changing Profiles of Service Sectors Used for Mental Health Care in the United States," *American Journal of Psychiatry* 163, no. 7 (July 2006): 1187–98, https://doi.org/10.1176/ajp.2006.163.7.1187.

29. Kaiser Family Foundation, "Professionally Active Physicians," January 2024, https://www.kff.org/other/state-indicator/total-active-physicians/?currentTimeframe=0&sortModel=%7B%22colId%22:%22Location%22,%22sort%22:%22asc%22%7D.

30. G. C. Alexander, J. Kurlander, and M. K. Wynia, "Physicians in Retainer ('Concierge') Practice: A National Survey of Physician, Patient, and Practice Characteristics," *Journal of General Internal Medicine* 20, no. 12 (December 2005): 1079–83, https://doi.org/10.1111/j.1525-1497.2005.0233.x; J. Altschuler, D. Margolius, T. Bodenheimer, and K. Grumbach, "Estimating a Reasonable Patient Panel Size for Primary Care Physicians with Team-Based Task Delegation," *Annals of Family Medicine* 10, no. 5 (September–October 2012): 396–400, https://doi.org/10.1370/afm.1400.

31. Association of American Medical Colleges, *Basic Science, Foundational Knowledge, and Pre-Clerkship Content: Average Number of Hours for Instruction/Assessment of Curriculum Subjects* (Washington, DC: Association of American Medical Colleges, 2012;

Association of American Medical Colleges, "Curriculum Reports," accessed June 7, 2024, https://www.aamc.org/data-reports/curriculum-reports/interactive-data/clinical -course-required-weeks-discipline; R. J. Choi, R. M. Betancourt, M. P. DeMarco, and K. D. W. Bream, "Medical Student Exposure to Integrated Behavioral Health," *Academic Psychiatry* 43, no. 2 (April 2019): 191–95, https://doi.org/10.1007/s40596-018-0936-0; M. P. DeMarco, R. M. Betancourt, K. M. Everard, and K. D. W. Bream, "Identifying Prevalence and Characteristics of Behavioral Health Education in Family Medicine Clerkships: A CERA Study," *Family Medicine* 50, no. 1 (January 2018): 36–40, https:// doi.org/10.22454/FamMed.2018.994360.

32. Association of American Medical Colleges, *Basic Science, Foundational Knowledge*.

33. Association of American Medical Colleges, "Curriculum Reports."

34. F. C. Dwamena, H. Laird-Fick, L. Freilich, D. D'Mello, J. Frey, A. Dasari, K. Grayson-Sneed, D. Solomon, and R. C. Smith, "Behavioral Health Problems in Medical Patients," *Journal of Clinical Outcomes Management* 21, no. 11 (November 2014): 497–505, https://www.mdedge.com/jcomjournal/article/147029/mental-health /behavioral-health-problems-medical-patients.

35. T. W. Croghan, M. Schoenbaum, C. D. Sherborne, and P. Koegel, "A Framework to Improve the Quality of Treatment for Depression in Primary Care," *Psychiatric Services* 57, no. 5 (May 2006): 623–30; Department of Health and Human Services, *Healthy People 2010: Understanding and Improving Health*, 2nd ed. (Washington, DC: US Government Printing Office, 2000); Dwamena et al., "Behavioral Health Problems"; L. Fisher and D. C. Ransom, "Developing a Strategy for Managing Behavioral Health Care within the Context of Primary Care," *Archives of Family Medicine* 6, no. 4 (July– August 1997): 324–33, https://doi.org/10.1001/archfami.6.4.324; Kathol et al., "Non-Traditional Mental Health"; Melek and Norris, *Chronic Conditions*.

36. Kessler et al., "Prevalence and Treatment"; P. S. Wang, S. Aguilar-Gaxiola, J. Alonso, M. C. Angermeyer, G. Borges, E. J. Bromet, R. Bruffaerts et al., "Use of Mental Health Services for Anxiety, Mood, and Substance Disorders in 17 Countries in the WHO World Mental Health Surveys," *Lancet* 370, no. 9590 (September 8, 2007): 841–50, https://doi.org/10.1016/S0140-6736(07)61414-7.

37. Kathol et al., "Non-Traditional Mental Health."

38. K. Stillwell, L. Pelkey, T. Platt, K. Nguyen, S. Monteith, A. Pinheiro, and E. D. Achtyes, "Survey of Primary Care Provider Comfort in Treating Psychiatric Patients in 2 Community Clinics: A Pilot Study," *Primary Care Companion for CNS Disorders* 24, no. 1 (2022): 21m03020, https://doi.org/10.4088/PCC.21m03020.

39. H. P. Chin, G. Guillermo, S. Prakken, and S. Eisendrath, "Psychiatric Training in Primary Care Medicine Residency Programs: A National Survey," *Psychosomatics* 41, no. 5 (September–October 2000): 412–17, https://doi.org/10.1176/appi.psy.41.5.412; H. Leigh, R. Mallios, and D. Stewart, "Teaching Psychiatry in Primary Care Residencies: Do Training Directors of Primary Care and Psychiatry See Eye to Eye?" *Academic Psychiatry* 32, no. 6 (November–December 2008): 504–9, https://doi.org/10.1176/appi .ap.32.6.504.

40. Chin et al., "Psychiatric Training."

41. E. H. Lin, W. J. Katon, G. E. Simon, M. Von Korff, T. M. Bush, C. M. Rutter, K. W. Saunders, and E. A. Walker, "Achieving Guidelines for the Treatment of Depres-

sion in Primary Care: Is Physician Education Enough?" *Medical Care* 35, no. 8 (August 1997): 831–42, https://doi.org/10.1097/00005650-199708000-00008.

42. S. Huo, T. A. Bruckner, G. L. Xiong, E. Cooper, A. Wade, A. B. Neikrug, J. P. Gagliardi, and R. McCarron, "Antidepressant Prescription Behavior among Primary Care Clinician Providers after an Interprofessional Primary Care Psychiatric Training Program," *Administration and Policy in Mental Health* 50, no. 6 (November 2023): 926–35, https://doi.org/10.1007/s10488-023-01290-x; UCI School of Medicine, "TNT PCP Fellowship Details," accessed June 7, 2024, https://medschool.uci.edu/educa tion/medical-education/cme/cme-tnt-fellowships/cme-tnt-pcp/cme-tnt-pcp-fellowship -details; A. B. Neikrug, A. Stehli, G. L. Xiong, S. Suo, K.-V. Le-Bucklin, W. Cant, and R. M. McCarron, "Train New Trainers Primary Care Psychiatry Fellowship-Optimizing Delivery of Behavioral Health Care through Training for Primary Care Providers," *Journal of Continuing Education in the Health Professions* 42, no. 2 (April 1, 2022): 105–14, https://doi.org/10.1097/CEH.0000000000000432.

43. F. W. Hafferty, "Beyond Curriculum Reform: Confronting Medicine's Hidden Curriculum," *Academic Medicine* 73, no. 4 (April 1998): 403–7, https://doi.org /10.1097/00001888-199804000-00013; J. T. H. Lam, M. D. Hanson, and M. A. T. Martimianakis, "Exploring the Socialization Experiences of Medical Students from Social Science and Humanities Backgrounds," *Academic Medicine* 95, no. 3 (March 2020): 401–10, https://doi.org/10.1097/ACM.0000000000002901; L. Shattock, H. Williamson, K. Caldwell, K. Anderson, and S. Peters, "'They've Just Got Symptoms without Science': Medical Trainees' Acquisition of Negative Attitudes towards Patients with Medically Unexplained Symptoms," *Patient Education and Counseling* 91, no. 2 (May 2013): 249–54, https://doi.org/1s0.1016/j.pec.2012.12.015; Starr, *Social Transformation of American Medicine*.

Chapter 3

1. B. Meier, "Opioid's Maker Hid Knowledge of Wide Abuse: Saw Early Evidence of Trouble, Report Says," *New York Times*, May 29, 2018, https://www.nytimes .com/2018/05/29/health/purdue-opioids-oxycontin.html.

2. National Academies of Sciences, Engineering, and Medicine, *Pain Management and the Opioid Epidemic: Balancing Societal and Individual Benefits and Risks of Prescription Opioid Use* (Washington, DC: National Academies Press, 2017).

3. Q. Chen, M. R. Larochelle, D. T. Weaver DT, A. P. Lietz, P. P. Mueller, S. Mercaldo, S. E. Wakeman et al., "Prevention of Prescription Opioid Misuse and Projected Overdose Deaths in the United States," *JAMA Network Open* 2, no. 2 (February 1, 2019): e187621, https://doi.org/10.1001/jamanetworkopen.2018.7621; Substance Abuse and Mental Health Services Administration, "2019–2020 National Survey on Drug Use and Health: Model-Based Prevalence Estimates (50 States and the District of Columbia)," December 29, 2021, https://www.samhsa.gov/data/report/2019-2020-ns duh-state-prevalence-estimates.

4. D. Dowell, T. M. Haegerich, and R. Chou, "CDC Guideline for Prescribing Opioids for Chronic Pain—United States," *Morbidity and Mortality Weekly Report* 65, no. 1 (March 18, 2016): 1–49, https://doi.org/10.15585/mmwr.rr6501e1; Chen et al., "Prevention of Prescription Opioid Misuse."

5. B. Han, W. M. Compton, C. Blanco, E. Crane, J. Lee, and C. M. Jones, "Prescription Opioid Use, Misuse, and Use Disorders in US Adults: 2015 National Survey on Drug Use and Health," *Annals of Internal Medicine* 167, no. 5 (September 5, 2017): 293–301, https://doi.org/10.7326/M17-0865.

6. R. C. Smith, C. Frank, J. C. Gardiner, L. Lamerato, and R. M. Rost, "Pilot Study of a Preliminary Criterion Standard for Prescription Opioid Misuse," *American Journal on Addictions* 19, no. 6 (November–December 2010): 523–28, https://doi.org/10.1111/j.1521-0391.2010.00084.x.

7. W. M. Compton and E. M. Wargo, "Prescription Drug Monitoring Programs: Promising Practices in Need of Refinement," *Annals of Internal Medicine* 168, no. 11 (June 5, 2018): 826–27, https://doi.org/10.7326/M18-0883; H. Wen, J. M. Hockenberry, P. J. Jeng, and Y. Bao, "Prescription Drug Monitoring Program Mandates: Impact on Opioid Prescribing and Related Hospital Use," *Health Affairs* 38, no. 9 (September 2019): 1550–56, https://doi.org/10.1377/hlthaff.2019.00103.

8. *Addressing the Opioid Crisis in America: Prevention, Treatment, and Recovery before the Senate Subcommittee on Labor, Health and Human Services, Education, and Related Agencies*, 115th Cong. (December 5, 2017) (statement of E. McCance-Katz, D. Houry, and F. Collins).

9. Talbott Recovery, "2015 Prescription Drug Abuse Statistics You Need to Know," accessed June 9, 2024, https://talbottcampus.com/resources/prescription-drug-abuse-statistics-2015/.

10. Talbott Recovery, "2015 Prescription Drug Abuse Statistics."

11. Talbott Recovery, "2015 Prescription Drug Abuse Statistics."

12. L. Manchikanti, S. Helm 2nd, B. Fellows, J. W. Janata, V. Pampati, J. S. Grider, and M. V. Boswell, "Opioid Epidemic in the United States," *Pain Physician* 15, no. 3 suppl. (July 2012): ES9–38, https://www.ncbi.nlm.nih.gov/pubmed/22786464.

13. B. Macy, *Dopesick: Dealers, Doctors, and the Drug Company That Addicted America* (New York: Little, Brown, 2018); Meier, "Opioid's Maker Hid Knowledge."

14. Manchikanti et al., "Opioid Epidemic in the United States."

15. D. K. Bäck, E. Tammaro, J. K. Lim, and S. E. Wakeman, "Massachusetts Medical Students Feel Unprepared to Treat Patients with Substance Use Disorder," *Journal of General Internal Medicine* 33, no. 3 (March 2018): 249–50, https://doi.org/10.1007/s11606-017-4192-x.

16. Manchikanti et al., "Opioid Epidemic in the United States."

17. G. T. Owen, A. W. Burton, C. M. Schade, and S. Passik, "Urine Drug Testing: Current Recommendations and Best Practices," *Pain Physician* 15, no. 3 suppl. (July 2012): ES119–33, https://www.ncbi.nlm.nih.gov/pubmed/22786451.

18. A. Lembke, "Why Doctors Prescribe Opioids to Known Opioid Abusers," *New England Journal of Medicine* 367, no. 17 (October 25, 2012): 1580–81, https://doi.org/10.1056/NEJMp1208498; Manchikanti et al., "Opioid Epidemic in the United

States"; M. D. Sullivan and J. C. Ballantyne, *The Right to Pain Relief and Other Deep Roots of the Opioid Epidemic* (New York: Oxford University Press, 2022).

19. Manchikanti et al., "Opioid Epidemic in the United States."

20. Dowell, Haegerich, and Chou, "CDC Guideline for Prescribing Opioids"; National Academies of Sciences, Engineering, and Medicine, *Pain Management.*

21. Dowell, Haegerich, and Chou, "CDC Guideline for Prescribing Opioids."

22. J. C. Ballantyne, M. D. Sullivan, and A. Kolodny, "Opioid Dependence vs. Addiction: A Distinction without a Difference?" *Archives of Internal Medicine* 172, no. 17 (September 24, 2012): 1342–43, https://doi.org/10.1001/archinternmed.2012.3212; C. Berna, R. J. Kulich, and J. P. Rathmell, "Tapering Long-Term Opioid Therapy in Chronic Noncancer Pain: Evidence and Recommendations for Everyday Practice," *Mayo Clinic Proceedings* 90, no. 6 (June 2015): 828–42, https://doi.org/10.1016/j.mayo cp.2015.04.003.

23. J. F. Scherrer, J. Salas, L. A. Copeland, E. M. Stock, B. K. Ahmedani, M. D. Sullivan, T. Burroughs, F. D. Schneider, K. K. Bucholz, and P. J. Lustman, "Prescription Opioid Duration, Dose, and Increased Risk of Depression in 3 Large Patient Populations," *Annals of Family Medicine* 14, no. 1 (January–February 2016): 54–62, https://doi.org/10.1370/afm.1885.

24. S. M. Silverman, "Opioid Induced Hyperalgesia: Clinical Implications for the Pain Practitioner," *Pain Physician* 12, no. 3 (May–June 2009): 679–84, http://www.ncbi.nlm.nih.gov/pubmed/19461836.

25. F. C. Dwamena, H. Laird-Fick, L. Freilich L, D. D'Mello, J. Frey, A. Dasari, K. Grayson-Sneed, D. Solomon, and R. C. Smith, "Behavioral Health Problems in Medical Patients," *Journal of Clinical Outcomes Management* 21, no. 11 (November 2014): 497–505, https://www.mdedge.com/jcomjournal/article/147029/mental-health/behavioral-health-problems-medical-patients.

26. A. Agnoli, G. Xing, D. J. Tancredi, E. Magnan, A. Jerant, and J. J. Fenton, "Association of Dose Tapering with Overdose or Mental Health Crisis among Patients Prescribed Long-Term Opioids," *JAMA* 326, no. 5 (August 3, 2021): 411–19, https://doi.org/10.1001/jama.2021.11013; P. O. Coffin and A. M. Barreveld, "Inherited Patients Taking Opioids for Chronic Pain—Considerations for Primary Care," *New England Journal of Medicine* 386, no. 7 (February 17, 2022): 611–13, https://doi.org/10.1056/NEJMp2115244; H. T. Neprash, M. Gaye, and M. L. Barnett, "Abrupt Discontinuation of Long-Term Opioid Therapy among Medicare Beneficiaries, 2012–2017," *Journal of General Internal Medicine* 36, no. 6 (June 2021): 1576–83, https://doi.org/10.1007/s11606-020-06402-z.

27. D. Dowell, T. Haegerich, and R. Chou, "No Shortcuts to Safer Opioid Prescribing," *New England Journal of Medicine* 380, no. 24 (June 13, 2019): 2285–87, https://doi.org/10.1056/NEJMp1904190; K. Kroenke, D. P. Alford, C. Argoff, B. Canlas, E. Covington, J. W. Frank, K. J. Haake et al., "Challenges with Implementing the Centers for Disease Control and Prevention Opioid Guideline: A Consensus Panel Report," *Pain Medicine* 20, no. 4 (April 1, 2019): 724–35, https://doi.org/10.1093/pm/pny307.

28. Ballantyne, Sullivan, and Kolodny, "Opioid Dependence vs. Addiction."

29. R. C. Smith, D. D'Mello, G. G. Osborn, L. Freilich, F. C. Dwamena, and H. Laird-Fick, *Essentials of Psychiatry in Primary Care: Behavioral Health in the Medical Setting* (New York: McGraw Hill Education, 2019).

30. J. A. Gordon, S. Avenevoli, and J. L. Pearson, "Suicide Prevention Research Priorities in Health Care," *JAMA Psychiatry* 77, no. 9 (September 1, 2020): 885–86, https://doi.org/10.1001/jamapsychiatry.2020.1042; M. F. Hogan and J. G. Grumet, "Suicide Prevention: An Emerging Priority for Health Care," *Health Affairs* 35, no. 6 (June 1, 2016): 1084–90, https://doi.org/10.1377/hlthaff.2015.1672.

31. M. Olfson, C. Blanco, M. Wall, S.-M. Liu, T. D. Saha, R. P. Pickering, and B. F. Grant, "National Trends in Suicide Attempts among Adults in the United States," *JAMA Psychiatry* 4, no. 11 (November 1, 2017): 1095–1103, https://doi.org/10.1001/jamapsychiatry.2017.2582.

32. 988 Suicide and Crisis Lifeline, accessed June 9, 2024, https://suicideprevention lifeline.org/; American Foundation for Suicide Prevention, "We Demand More Funding for 988 for Mental Health, accessed June 9, 2024, https://moreformentalhealth.org /funding.htm.

33. U. Lewitzka, C. Sauer, M. Bauer, and W. Felber, "Are National Suicide Prevention Programs Effective? A Comparison of 4 Verum and 4 Control Countries over 30 Years," *BMC Psychiatry* 19, no. 1 (May 23, 2019): 158, https://doi.org/10.1186/s12888 -019-2147-y.

34. Hogan and Grumet, "Suicide Prevention"; R. M. McCarron, E. R. Vanderlip, and J. Rado, "Depression," *Annals of Internal Medicine* 165, no. 7 (October 4, 2016): ITC49–64, https://doi.org/10.7326/AITC201610040.

35. C. Crump, A. C. Edwards, K. S. Kendler, J. Sundquist, and K. Sundquist, "Healthcare Utilisation Prior to Suicide in Persons with Alcohol Use Disorder: National Cohort and Nested Case-Control Study," *British Journal of Psychiatry* 217, no. 6 (December 2020): 710–16, https://doi.org/10.1192/bjp.2020.122.

36. Hogan and Grumet, "Suicide Prevention."

37. Association of American Medical Colleges, *Basic Science, Foundational Knowledge, and Pre-Clerkship Content: Average Number of Hours for Instruction/Assessment of Curriculum Subjects* (Washington, DC: Association of American Medical Colleges, 2012); Association of American Medical Colleges, "Curriculum Reports," accessed June 7, 2024, https://www.aamc.org/data-reports/curriculum-reports/interactive-data/clinical -course-required-weeks-discipline; R. J. Choi, R. M. Betancourt, M. P. DeMarco, and K. D. W. Bream, "Medical Student Exposure to Integrated Behavioral Health," *Academic Psychiatry* 43, no. 2 (April 2019): 191–95, https://doi.org/10.1007/s40596-018-0936-0; M. P. DeMarco, R. M. Betancourt, K. M. Everard, and K. D. W. Bream, "Identifying Prevalence and Characteristics of Behavioral Health Education in Family Medicine Clerkships: A CERA Study," *Family Medicine* 50, no. 1 (January 2018): 36–40, https://doi.org/10.22454/FamMed.2018.994360.

38. American Psychiatric Association, *Diagnostic and Statistical Manual of Mental Disorders: DSM-5*, 5th ed. (Washington, DC: American Psychiatric Association, 2013).

39. Dwamena et al., "Behavioral Health Problems."

40. N. Panchal, H. Saunders, R. Rudowitz, and C. Cox, "The Implications of COVID-19 for Mental Health and Substance Use," Kaiser Family Foundation, March

20, 2023, https://www.kff.org/coronavirus-covid-19/issue-brief/the-implications-of-co vid-19-for-mental-health-and-substance-use/.

41. M. É. Czeisler, R. I. Lane, E. Petrosky, J. F. Wiley, A. Christensen, R. Njai, M. D. Weaver et al., "Mental Health, Substance Use, and Suicidal Ideation during the COVID-19 Pandemic—United States, June 24–30, 2020," *Morbidity and Mortality Weekly Report* 69, no. 32 (August 14, 2020): 1049–57, https://doi.org/10.15585/mmwr .mm6932a1.

42. N. Racine, B. A. McArthur, J. E. Cooke, R. Eirich, J. Zhu, and S. Madigan, "Global Prevalence of Depressive and Anxiety Symptoms in Children and Adolescents during COVID-19: A Meta-Analysis," *JAMA Pediatrics* 175, no. 11 (November 1, 2021): 1142–50, https://doi.org/10.1001/jamapediatrics.2021.2482.

43. National Center for Health Statistics, "Anxiety and Depression," Centers for Disease Control and Prevention, updated May 16, 2024, https://www.cdc.gov/nchs /covid19/pulse/mental-health.htm.

44. Center for Disease Control and Prevention, "Coronavirus Disease, Coping with Stress," 2020; B. Pfefferbaum and C. S. North, "Mental Health and the Covid-19 Pandemic," *New England Journal of Medicine* 383, no. 6 (August 6, 2020): 510–12, https:// doi.org/10.1056/NEJMp2008017; D. Vigo S. Patten, K. Pajer, M. Krausz, S. Taylor, B. Rush, G. Raviola, S. Saxena, G. Thornicroft, and L. N. Yatham, "Mental Health of Communities during the COVID-19 Pandemic," *Canadian Journal of Psychiatry* 65, no. 10 (October 2020): 681–87, https://doi.org/10.1177/0706743720926676.

45. R. Pearl, *Uncaring: How the Culture of Medicine Kills Doctors and Patients* (New York: PublicAffairs, 2021).

46. K. L. Syme and E. H. Hagen, "Mental Health Is Biological Health: Why Tackling 'Diseases of the Mind' Is an Imperative for Biological Anthropology in the 21st Century," *American Journal of Physical Anthropology* 171, suppl. 70 (May 2020): 87–117, https://doi.org/10.1002/ajpa.23965.

47. Marshall Protocol Knowledge Base, "The Ten Leading Causes of Death in the United States in 1900 and 1997," accessed June 9, 2024, https://www.bing.com/images /search?view=detailV2&id=A4BA55922CFF3B4CD8461520D3DC25DC5BB87EC3 &thid=OIP.SG-5a3mk00sugRbAuByvdwHaH_&mediaurl=https%3A%2F%2Fmpkb .org%2F_media%2Fhome%2Fpathogenesis%2Fmortality.gif&exph=432&expw=400&q =chronic+disease+prevalence+us+graphics&selectedindex=0&qpvt=chronic+disease+preval ence+us+graphics&ajaxhist=0&vt=0.

48. Statista, "Distribution of the 10 Leading Causes of Death in the United States in 2022," 2024, https://www.statista.com/statistics/248619/leading-causes-of-death-in -the-us/.

49. Centers for Disease Control and Prevention, "About Chronic Diseases," May 15, 2024, https://www.cdc.gov/chronic-disease/about/?CDC_AAref_Val=https://www.cdc .gov/chronicdisease/about/index.htm.

50. B. G. Druss and E. R. Walker, "Mental Disorders and Medical Comorbidity," *Synthesis Project: Research Synthesis Report*, no. 21 (February 2011): 1–26, https:// pubmed.ncbi.nlm.nih.gov/21650091/.

51. R. Kathol, S. Sargent, S. Melek, L. Sacks, and K. Patel, "Non-Traditional Mental Health and Substance Use Disorder Services as a Core Part of Health in CINs

and ACOs," *Clinical Integration: Population Health and Accountable Care*, 3rd ed., ed. K. Yale, T. A. Raskauskas, J. Bohn, and C. Konschak, 380–425 (Virginia Beach, VA: Convergent, 2015); V. Patel and S. Chatterji, "Integrating Mental Health in Care for Noncommunicable Diseases: An Imperative for Person-Centered Care," *Health Affairs* 34, no. 9 (September 2015): 1498–1505, https://doi.org/10.1377/hlthaff.2015.0791.

52. N. C. Momen, O. Plana-Ripoll, A. Agerbo, M. K. Christensen, K. M. Iburg, T. M. Laursen, P. B. Mortensen et al., "Mortality Associated with Mental Disorders and Comorbid General Medical Conditions," *JAMA Psychiatry* 79, no. 5 (May 1, 2022): 444–53, https://doi.org/10.1001/jamapsychiatry.2022.0347.

53. P. Frank, G. D. Batty, J. Pentti, M. Jokela, L. Poole, J. Ervasti, J. Vahtera, G. Lewis, A. Steptoe, and M. Kivimäki, "Association between Depression and Physical Conditions Requiring Hospitalization," *JAMA Psychiatry* 80, no. 7 (July 1, 2023), https://doi.org/10.1001/jamapsychiatry.2023.0777; W. M. Hooten, "Chronic Pain and Mental Health Disorders: Shared Neural Mechanisms, Epidemiology, and Treatment," *Mayo Clinic Proceedings* 91, no. 7 (July 2016): 955–70, https://doi.org/10.1016/j.mayo cp.2016.04.029.

54. Momen et al., "Association between Mental Disorders"; K. M. Scott, C. Lim, A. Al-Hamzawi, R. Bruffaerts, J. M. Caldas-de-Almeida, S. Florescu et al., "Association of Mental Disorders with Subsequent Chronic Physical Conditions: World Mental Health Surveys from 17 Countries," *JAMA Psychiatry* 73, no. 2 (February 2016): 150–58, https://doi.org/10.1001/jamapsychiatry.2015.2688.

55. E. L. Harshfield, L. Pennells, J. E. Schwartz, P. Willeit, S. Kaptoge, S. Bell, J. A. Shaffer, et al., "Association between Depressive Symptoms and Incident Cardiovascular Diseases," *JAMA* 324, no. 23 (December 15, 2020): 2396–2405, https://doi .org/10.1001/jama.2020.23068; S. Rajan, M. McKee, S. Rangarajan, S. Bangdiwala, A. Rosengren, R. Gupta, V. R. Kutty et al., "Association of Symptoms of Depression with Cardiovascular Disease and Mortality in Low-, Middle-, and High-Income Countries," *JAMA Psychiatry* 77, no. 10 (October 1, 2020): 1052–63, https://doi.org/10.1001 /jamapsychiatry.2020.1351.

56. J. Wertz, A. Caspi, A. Ambler, J. Broadbent, R. J. Hancox, H. Harrington, S. Hogan et al., "Association of History of Psychopathology with Accelerated Aging at Midlife," *JAMA Psychiatry* 78, no. 5 (May 1, 2021): 530–39, https://doi.org/10.1001 /jamapsychiatry.2020.4626.

57. Hooten, "Chronic Pain."

58. Druss and Walker, "Mental Disorders and Medical Comorbidity"; Hooten, "Chronic Pain"; Patel and Chatterji, "Integrating Mental Health."

59. J. Walker, A. Mulick, N. Magill, S. Symeonides, C. Gourley, K. Burke, A. Belot et al., "Major Depression and Survival in People with Cancer," *Psychosomatic Medicine* 83, no. 5 (June 1, 2021): 410–16, https://doi.org/10.1097/PSY.0000000000000942.

60. J. J. Gallo, S. Hwang, J. H. Joo JH, H. R. Bogner, K. H. Morales, M. L. Bruce, C. F. Reynolds 3rd, "Multimorbidity, Depression, and Mortality in Primary Care: Randomized Clinical Trial of an Evidence-Based Depression Care Management Program on Mortality Risk," *Journal of General Internal Medicine* 31, no. 4 (April 2016): 380–86, https://doi.org/10.1007/s11606-015-3524-y; J. F. van Eck van der Sluijs, H. Castelijns, V. Eijsbroek, C. A. T. Rijnders, H. W. J. van Marwijk, and C. M. van der Feltz-Cornelis,

"Illness Burden and Physical Outcomes Associated with Collaborative Care in Patients with Comorbid Depressive Disorder in Chronic Medical Conditions: A Systematic Review and Meta-Analysis," *General Hospital Psychiatry* 50 (January–February 2018): 1–14, https://doi.org/10.1016/j.genhosppsych.2017.08.003.

61. Gallo et al., "Multimorbidity, Depression, and Mortality"; van Eck van der Sluijs et al., "Illness Burden and Physical Outcomes."

62. Druss and Walker, "Mental Disorders and Medical Comorbidity"; Kathol, Sargent et al., "Non-Traditional Mental Health."

63. S. A. Frankel, J. A. Bourgeois, and P. Erdberg, *Comprehensive Care for Complex Patients: The Medical-Psychiatric Coordinating Physician Model* (Cambridge, UK: Cambridge University Press, 2013); S. A. Frankel, S. D. Thurber, and J. A. Bourgeois, *Complexity in Health Care: A Paradigm Shift for Clinical Practice* (Cham, Switzerland: Springer, 2023); R. G. Kathol, M. Butler, D. D. McAlpine, and R. L. Kane, "Barriers to Physical and Mental Condition Integrated Service Delivery," *Psychosomatic Medicine* 72, no. 6 (July 2010): 511–18, https://doi.org/10.1097/PSY.0b013e3181e2c4a0; Kathol, Sargent et al., "Non-Traditional Mental Health."

64. P. L. Remington, R. C. Brownson, and M. V. Wegner (eds.), *Chronic Disease Epidemiology and Control*, 3rd ed. (Washington, DC: American Public Health Association, 2010).

65. Partnership to Fight Chronic Disease, "The Growing Crisis of Chronic Disease in the United States," accessed June 9, 2024, https://www.fightchronicdisease.org/sites/default/files/docs/GrowingCrisisofChronicDiseaseintheUSfactsheet_81009.pdf.

66. Pearl, *Uncaring*.

67. M. McKillop and D. A. Lieberman, *The Impact of Chronic Underfunding on America's Public Health System: Trends, Risks, and Recommendations 2023* (Washington, DC: Trust for America's Health, June 2023), https://www.tfah.org/wp-content/uploads/2023/06/TFAH-2023-PublicHealthFundingFINALc.pdf.

68. Z. A. Marcum, M. A. Sevick, and S. M. Handler, "Medication Nonadherence: A Diagnosable and Treatable Medical Condition," *JAMA* 309, no. 20 (May 22, 2013): 2105–6, https://doi.org/10.1001/jama.2013.4638.

69. M. T. Brown and J. K. Bussell, "Medication Adherence: WHO Cares?" *Mayo Clinic Proceedings* 86, no. 4 (April 2011): 304–14, https://doi.org/10.4065/mcp.2010.0575; Marcum, Sevick, and Handler, "Medication Nonadherence."

70. H. Al-Noumani, J.-R. Wu, D. Barksdale, G. Sherwood, E. AlKhasawneh, and G. Knafl, "Health Beliefs and Medication Adherence in Patients with Hypertension: A Systematic Review of Quantitative Studies," *Patient Education and Counseling* 102, no. 6 (June 2019): 1045–56, https://doi.org/10.1016/j.pec.2019.02.022.

71. J. M. Hensel, V. H. Taylor, K. Fung, C. de Oliveira, and S. N. Vigod, "Unique Characteristics of High-Cost Users of Medical Care with Comorbid Mental Illness or Addiction in a Population-Based Cohort," *Psychosomatics* 59, no. 2 (March–April 2018): 135–43, https://doi.org/10.1016/j.psym.2017.10.005; S. Melek, M. Halford, and D. Perlman, *Depression Treatment: The Impact of Treatment Persistence on Total Healthcare Costs*, Milliman Research Report (Denver, CO: Milliman, June 2012), https://www.milliman.com/-/media/milliman/importedfiles/uploadedfiles/insight/health-published/pdfs/depression-treatment.ashx; S. Melek and D. Norris, *Chronic Conditions and*

Comorbid Psychological Disorders, Milliman Research Report (Seattle, WA: Milliman, July 2008), https://www.cbhc.org/wp-content/uploads/2015/11/chronic-conditions -and-comorbid-RR07-01-08.pdf; S. P. Melek, D. T. Norris, and J. Paulus, *Economic Impact of Integrated Medical-Behavioral Healthcare: Implications for Psychiatry*, Milliman American Psychiatric Association Report (Denver, CO: Milliman, April 2014), https:// www.coloradocoalition.org/sites/default/files/2017-01/milliaman-apa-economicimpact ofintegratedmedicalbehavioralhealthcare2014.pdf.

72. Druss and Walker, "Mental Disorders and Medical Comorbidity."

73. L. A. Graham, M. T. Hawn, E. A. Dasinger, S. J. Baker, B. S. Oriel, T. S. Wahl, J. S. Richman et al., "Psychosocial Determinants of Readmission after Surgery," *Medical Care* 59, no. 10 (October 1, 2021): 864–71, https://doi.org/10.1097 /MLR.0000000000001600; Melek and Norris, *Chronic Conditions*.

74. Melek and Norris, *Chronic Conditions*.

75. Melek and Norris, *Chronic Conditions*.

76. Melek, Norris, and Paulus, *Economic Impact*.

77. Department of Health and Human Services, "HHS FY 2018 Budget in Brief," National Institutes of Health, 2017.

78. Brown and Bussell, "Medication Adherence"; Marcum, Sevick, and Handler, "Medication Nonadherence."

79. M. Hartman, A. B. Martin, L. Whittle, and A. Catlin, "National Health Care Spending in 2022: Growth Similar to Prepandemic Rates," *Health Affairs* 43, no. 1 (January 2024): 6–17, https://doi.org/10.1377/hlthaff.2023.01360; A. B. Martin, M. Hartman, D. Lassman, and A. Catlin, "National Health Care Spending in 2019: Steady Growth for the Fourth Consecutive Year," *Health Affairs* 40, no. 1 (January 2021): 14–21, https://doi.org/10.1377/hlthaff.2020.02022; Partnership to Fight Chronic Disease, "Growing Crisis of Chronic Disease."

80. Partnership to Fight Chronic Disease, "Growing Crisis of Chronic Disease."

81. D. Khullar, Y. Zhang, and R. Kaushal, "Potentially Preventable Spending among High-Cost Medicare Patients: Implications for Healthcare Delivery," *Journal of General Internal Medicine* 35, no. 10 (October 2020): 2845–52, https://doi.org/10.1007 /s11606-020-05691-8; J. J. Zhang, M. B. Rothberg, A. D. Misra-Hebert, N. M. Gupta, and G. B. Taksler, "Assessment of Physician Priorities in Delivery of Preventive Care," *JAMA Network Open* 3, no. 7 (July 1, 2020): e2011677, https://doi.org/10.1001/jama networkopen.2020.11677.

Chapter 4

1. F. H. Garrison, *An Introduction to the History of Medicine: With Medical Chronology, Suggestions for Study and Bibliographic Data*, 4th ed. (Philadelphia: W. B. Saunders, 1929); R. Porter, *The Greatest Benefit to Mankind: A Medical History of Humanity* (New York: W. W. Norton, 2009).

2. Garrison, *Introduction to the History*; Porter, *Greatest Benefit to Mankind*; D. Schneider, *The Invention of Surgery: History of Modern Medicine: From the Renaissance to the Implant Revolution* (New York: Pegasus Books, 2020).

3. S. Browne and M. Burton, *The History of Psychiatry: Important Figures and Developments* (Scotts Valley, CA: CreateSpace Independent Publishing Platform, 2015); Porter, *Greatest Benefit to Mankind.*

4. Garrison, *Introduction to the History*; R. Porter, "What Is Disease?" in *Cambridge History of Medicine*, ed. R. Porter, 71–102 (Cambridge, UK: Cambridge University Press, 2011).

5. Porter, *Greatest Benefit to Mankind.*

6. Porter, "What Is Disease?"

7. Porter, "What Is Disease?"

8. Porter, *Greatest Benefit to Mankind.*

9. Browne and Burton, *History of Psychiatry*; Garrison, *Introduction to the History.*

10. Garrison, *Introduction to the History.*

11. Garrison, *Introduction to the History.*

12. A. G. Carmichael and R. M. Ratzan (eds.), *Medicine: A Treasury of Art and Literature* (New York: Hugh Lauter Levin, 1991.

13. Browne and Burton, *History of Psychiatry.*

14. Porter, *Greatest Benefit to Mankind.*

15. R. Porter, "Mental Illness," in *Cambridge History of Medicine*, ed. R. Porter, 238–59 (Cambridge, UK: Cambridge University Press, 2011).

16. Porter, "Mental Illness."

17. Porter, *Greatest Benefit to Mankind.*

18. Porter, *Greatest Benefit to Mankind*; Porter, "What Is Disease?"

19. Porter, *Greatest Benefit to Mankind.*

20. Porter, *Greatest Benefit to Mankind.*

21. Garrison, *Introduction to the History*; Schneider, *Invention of Surgery.*

22. V. Nutton, "The Rise of Medicine," in *The Cambridge History of Medicine*, ed. R. Porter, 46–70 (Cambridge, UK: Cambridge University Press, 2011).

23. Porter, *Greatest Benefit to Mankind.*

24. M. Friedman and G. W. Friedland, *Medicine's 10 Greatest Discoveries* (New Haven, CT: Yale University Press, 1998).

25. Porter, *Greatest Benefit to Mankind.*

26. Garrison, *Introduction to the History*; Porter, *Greatest Benefit to Mankind.*

27. Porter, *Greatest Benefit to Mankind.*

28. Garrison, *Introduction to the History*; Porter, *Greatest Benefit to Mankind.*

29. Nutton, "Rise of Medicine"; Porter, *Greatest Benefit to Mankind.*

30. Friedman and Friedland, *Medicine's 10 Greatest Discoveries.*

31. Porter, *Greatest Benefit to Mankind.*

32. Friedman and Friedland, *Medicine's 10 Greatest Discoveries.*

33. Friedman and Friedland, *Medicine's 10 Greatest Discoveries*; S. K. Ghosh, "Human Cadaveric Dissection: A Historical Account from Ancient Greece to the Modern Era," *Anatomy and Cell Biology* 48, no. 3 (September 2015): 153–69, https://doi .org/10.5115/acb.2015.48.3.153; R. Porter, "Medical Science," in *Cambridge History of Medicine*, ed. R. Porter, 136–75 (Cambridge, UK: Cambridge University Press, 2011); Schneider, *Invention of Surgery*; K. Walker, *The Story of Medicine* (New York: Oxford University Press, 1955).

34. Porter, "Medical Science."

35. G. L. Engel, "The Need for a New Medical Model: A Challenge for Biomedicine," *Science* 196, no. 4286 (April 8, 1977): 129–36, https://doi.org/10.1126/science.847460.

36. Garrison, *Introduction to the History.*

37. Porter, "Medical Science."

38. Friedman and Friedland, *Medicine's 10 Greatest Discoveries*; Schneider, *Invention of Surgery.*

39. Ghosh, "Human Cadaveric Dissection."

40. Friedman and Friedland, *Medicine's 10 Greatest Discoveries*; Ghosh, "Human Cadaveric Dissection"; S. B. Nuland, *Doctors: The Biography of Medicine* (New York: Vintage Books, 1988).

41. Friedman and Friedland, *Medicine's 10 Greatest Discoveries.*

42. R. Wilkins (ed.), *The Doctor's Quotation Book: A Medical Miscellany* (New York: Barnes and Noble, 1991).

43. Nuland, *Doctors*; Schneider, *Invention of Surgery.*

44. Friedman and Friedland, *Medicine's 10 Greatest Discoveries.*

45. I. M. L. Donaldson, "Andreae Vesalii Bruxellensis Icones Anatomicae: Part 1," *Journal of the Royal College of Physicians in Edinburgh* 42, no. 2 (June 2012): 184–86, https://doi.org/10.4997/JRCPE.2012.220; Friedman and Friedland, *Medicine's 10 Greatest Discoveries*; F. Guerra, "The Identity of the Artists Involved in Vesalius's *Fabrica* 1543," *Medical History* 13, no. 1 (January 1969): 37–50, https://doi.org/10.1017/s0025727300013934.

46. Friedman and Friedland, *Medicine's 10 Greatest Discoveries*; Ghosh, "Human Cadaveric Dissection"; Schneider, *Invention of Surgery.*

47. Friedman and Friedland, *Medicine's 10 Greatest Discoveries.*

48. Ghosh, "Human Cadaveric Dissection."

49. Ghosh, "Human Cadaveric Dissection."

50. Rembrandt van Rijn, *The Anatomy Lesson of Dr. Nicolaes Tulp*, Mauritshuis, 1632, https://www.mauritshuis.nl/en/our-collection/artworks/146-the-anatomy-lesson-of-dr-nicolaes-tulp/.

51. Ghosh, "Human Cadaveric Dissection"; van Rijn, *Anatomy Lesson.*

52. F. F. Ijpma, N. E. Middelkoop, and T. M. van Gulik, "Rembrandt's *Anatomy Lesson of Dr. Deijman* of 1656 Dissected," *Neurosurgery* 73, no. 3 (September 2013): 381–85, https://doi.org/10.1227/01.neu.0000430284.62810.4b; J. P. W. F. Lakke, "Autopsy Practises for Brain Dissections and Rembrandt's *Anatomy Lesson of Dr. Deijman*," *Journal of the History of the Neurosciences* 7, no. 2 (August 1998): 101–7, https://doi.org/10.1076/jhin.7.2.101.1869.

53. Friedman and Friedland, *Medicine's 10 Greatest Discoveries*; Porter, "Medical Science."

54. Porter, "Medical Science."

55. Friedman and Friedland, *Medicine's 10 Greatest Discoveries*; Porter, "Medical Science."

56. Porter, "Medical Science"; Porter, "What Is Disease?"

57. Porter, "Medical Science."

58. Schneider, *Invention of Surgery*.

59. M. Foucault, *The Birth of the Clinic: An Archeology of Medical Perception*, trans. A. M. S. Smith (New York: Vintage Books, 1973).

Chapter 5

1. *Merriam-Webster*, "Subconscious," accessed June 14, 2024, https://www.mer riam-webster.com/dictionary/subconscious.

2. R. Porter, *The Greatest Benefit to Mankind: A Medical History of Humanity* (New York: W. W. Norton, 2009); R. Porter, "What Is Disease?" in *Cambridge History of Medicine*, ed. R. Porter, 71–102 (Cambridge, UK: Cambridge University Press, 2011).

3. Porter, *Greatest Benefit to Mankind*; R. Porter, "Medical Science," in *Cambridge History of Medicine*, ed. R. Porter, 136–75 (Cambridge, UK: Cambridge University Press, 2011); M. D. Sullivan, *The Patient as Agent of Health and Health Care* (New York: Oxford University Press, 2017).

4. G. Duncan, "Mind-Body Dualism and the Biopsychosocial Model of Pain: What Did Descartes Really Say?" *Journal of Medicine and Philosophy* 25, no. 4 (August 2000): 485–513, https://doi.org/10.1076/0360-5310(200008)25:4;1-A;FT485; N. Mehta, "Mind-Body Dualism: A Critique from a Health Perspective," *Mens Sana Monographs* 9, no. 1 (January 2011): 202–9, http://www.ncbi.nlm.nih.gov/pubmed/21694971; G. Ryle, "Descartes' Myth," in *The Concept of Mind*, 11–24 (London: Hutchinson's University Library, 1949); R. Young, "The Mind-Body Problem," in *Companion to the History of Modern Science*, ed. R. C. Olby, G. N. Cantor, J. R. R. Christie, and M. J. S. Hodge, 702–11 (London: Routledge, 1990).

5. F. Capra and P. Luisi, *The Systems View of Life: A Unifying Vision* (Cambridge, UK: Cambridge University Press, 2014); Young, "Mind-Body Problem."

6. Sullivan, *Patient as Agent of Health*; C. Taylor, *Sources of the Self: The Making of the Modern Identity* (Cambridge, MA: Harvard University Press, 1989).

7. Young, "Mind-Body Problem."

8. Porter, *Greatest Benefit to Mankind*; Ryle, "Descartes' Myth."

9. Mehta, "Mind-Body Dualism"; Sullivan, *Patient as Agent of Health*.

10. Sullivan, *Patient as Agent of Health*; Taylor, *Sources of the Self*.

11. Porter, *Greatest Benefit to Mankind*; Sullivan, *Patient as Agent of Health*.

12. Sullivan, *Patient as Agent of Health*.

13. Sullivan, *Patient as Agent of Health*; Taylor, *Sources of the Self*.

14. Porter, *Greatest Benefit to Mankind*.

15. T. M. Brown, "Cartesian Dualism and Psychosomatics," *Psychosomatics* 30, no. 3 (Summer 1989): 322–31, https://doi.org/10.1016/S0033-3182(89)72280-5; F. H. Garrison, *An Introduction to the History of Medicine: With Medical Chronology, Suggestions for Study and Bibliographic Data*, 4th ed. (Philadelphia: W. B. Saunders, 1929); Porter, "Medical Science"; D. Schneider, *The Invention of Surgery: History of Modern Medicine: From the Renaissance to the Implant Revolution* (New York: Pegasus Books, 2020).

16. Porter, *Greatest Benefit to Mankind*; Porter, "Medical Science"; Porter, "What Is Disease?"

17. E. H. Bradley and L. A. Tayor, *The American Health Care Paradox—Why Spending More Is Getting Us Less* (New York: PublicAffairs, 2013); M. Foucault, *The Birth of the Clinic: An Archeology of Medical Perception*, trans. A. M. S. Smith (New York: Vintage Books, 1973); M. Friedman and G. W. Friedland, *Medicine's 10 Greatest Discoveries* (New Haven, CT: Yale University Press, 1998); A. Marom, "The Birth, Death, and Renaissance (?) of Dissection: A Critique of Anatomy Teaching with—or without—the Human Body," *Academic Medicine* 95, no. 7 (July 2020): 999–1005, https://doi .org/10.1097/ACM.0000000000003090; Porter, *Greatest Benefit to Mankind*; Porter, "Medical Science"; M. Sullivan, "In What Sense Is Contemporary Medicine Dualistic?" *Culture, Medicine and Psychiatry* 10, no. 4 (December 1986): 331–50, https://doi .org/10.1007/BF00049269.

18. Friedman and Friedland, *Medicine's 10 Greatest Discoveries*.

19. S. B. Nuland, *Doctors: The Biography of Medicine* (New York: Vintage Books, 1988).

20. Garrison, *Introduction to the History*; J. B. Morgagni and W. Cooke, *The Seats and Causes of Disease, Investigated by Anatomy, Containing a Great Variety of Dissections, and Accompanied with Remarks* (Boston: Wells and Lilly, 1824), https://archive.org/details /seatscausesofdis002morg/page/n7/mode/2up; Nuland, *Doctors*; Porter, *Greatest Benefit to Mankind*; Porter, "Medical Science."

21. Nuland, *Doctors*; F. Zampieri, A. Zanatta, and G. Thiene, "An Etymological 'Autopsy' of Morgagni's Title: *De Sedibus et Causis Morborum per Anatomen Indagatis* (1761)," *Human Pathology* 45, no. 1 (January 2014): 12–16, https://doi.org/10.1016/j .humpath.2013.04.019.

22. Garrison, *Introduction to the History*; Porter, *Greatest Benefit to Mankind*.

23. Nuland, *Doctors*.

24. Morgagni and Cooke, *Seats and Causes of Disease*.

25. Foucault, *Birth of the Clinic*; Garrison, *Introduction to the History*; Nuland, *Doctors*; Porter, *Greatest Benefit to Mankind*; Porter, "Medical Science"; Sullivan, "In What Sense."

26. Nuland, *Doctors*.

27. S. Mukherjee, *Song of the Cell: An Exploration of Medicine and the New Human* (New York: Scribner, 2023).

28. Foucault, *Birth of the Clinic*.

29. Nuland, *Doctors*; Sullivan, "In What Sense."

30. Foucault, *Birth of the Clinic*.

31. N. G. Hale Jr., *Freud and the Americans: The Beginnings of Psychoanalysis in the United States, 1876–1917* (New York: Oxford University Press, 1971); Porter, "Medical Science"; S. J. Reiser, *Medicine and the Reign of Technology* (Cambridge, UK: Cambridge University Press, 1978); Schneider, *Invention of Surgery*; E. Shorter, "Primary Care," in *Cambridge History of Medicine*, ed. R. Porter, 103–35 (Cambridge, UK: Cambridge University Press, 2011).

32. Sullivan, "In What Sense."

33. Nuland, *Doctors*; Porter, "Medical Science."

34. Sullivan, "In What Sense."

35. Mukherjee, *Song of the Cell*; Nuland, *Doctors*.

36. Schneider, *Invention of Surgery*.

37. Garrison, *Introduction to the History*; Porter, *Greatest Benefit to Mankind*.

38. Porter, "Medical Science"; Schneider, *Invention of Surgery*; Sullivan, *Patient as Agent of Health*.

39. Porter, "Medical Science."

40. Sullivan, *Patient as Agent of Health*.

41. A. H. Fortin VI, F. C. Dwamena, R. M. Frankel, B. L. Lepisto, and R. C. Smith, *Smith's Patient-Centered Interviewing: An Evidence-Based Method*, 4th ed. (New York: McGraw-Hill Education, 2018); J. L. Jameson, A. S. Fauci, D. L. Kasper, S. L. Hauser, D. L. Longo, and J. Loscalzo (eds.), *Harrison's Principles of Internal Medicine*, 20th ed. (New York: McGraw-Hill Education, 2018).

42. A. S. Detsky, "Learning the Art and Science of Diagnosis," *JAMA* 327, no. 18 (May 10, 2022): 1759–60, https://doi.org/10.1001/jama.2022.4650; Fortin et al., *Smith's Patient-Centered Interviewing*.

43. Association of American Medical Colleges, *Basic Science, Foundational Knowledge, and Pre-Clerkship Content: Average Number of Hours for Instruction/Assessment of Curriculum Subjects* (Washington, DC: Association of American Medical Colleges, 2012); Association of American Medical Colleges, "Curriculum Reports," accessed June 7, 2024, https://www.aamc.org/data-reports/curriculum-reports/interactive-data/clinical-course -required-weeks-discipline.

44. Sullivan, "In What Sense."

45. A. Dua, P. D. Sutphin, M. J. Siedner, and J. Moran, "Case 16-2021: A 37-Year-Old Woman with Abdominal Pain and Aortic Dilatation," *New England Journal of Medicine* 384, no. 21 (May 27, 2021): 2054–63, https://doi.org/10.1056/NEJMcpc2100278.

46. R. B. Bean (comp.), *Sir William Osler Aphorisms: From His Bedside Teachings and Writings*, ed. W. B. Bean (Springfield, IL: C. C. Thomas, 1961).

47. W. Osler, *The Principles and Practice of Medicine—Designed for the Use of Practitioners and Students of Medicine*, 8th ed. (New York: D. Appleton, 1912); S. Johnson, *Extra Life: A Short History of Living Longer* (New York: Riverhead Books, 2021).

48. R. Wilkins (ed.), *The Doctor's Quotation Book: A Medical Miscellany* (New York: Barnes and Noble Books, 1991).

49. Shorter, "Primary Care."

50. Shorter, "Primary Care."

51. Schneider, *Invention of Surgery*; Shorter, "Primary Care."

52. Schneider, *Invention of Surgery*.

53. Porter, *Greatest Benefit to Mankind*.

54. Agency for Healthcare Research and Quality, "The Number of Practicing Primary Care Physicians in the United States: Primary Care Workforce Facts and Stats No. 1," last reviewed February 2024, https://www.ahrq.gov/sites/default/files/publications /files/pcwork1.pdf; Porter, *Greatest Benefit to Mankind*; P. Starr, *The Social Transformation of American Medicine* (New York: Basic Books, 1982).

55. National Center for Health Statistics, *Health United States, 2015: With Special Feature on Racial and Ethnic Health Disparities* (Washington, DC: US Department of

Health and Human Services, May 2016), https://www.cdc.gov/nchs/data/hus/hus15
.pdf; R. Crowley, S. Mathew, D. Hilden, and Health and Public Policy Committee of
the American College of Physicians, "Modernizing the United States' Public Health
Infrastructure: A Position Paper from the American College of Physicians," *Annals of
Internal Medicine* 176, no. 8 (August 2023): 1089–91, https://doi.org/10.7326/M23
-0670; Johnson, *Extra Life*.

   56. S. Capewell, C. E. Morrison, and J. J. McMurray, "Contribution of Modern
Cardiovascular Treatment and Risk Factor Changes to the Decline in Coronary Heart
Disease Mortality in Scotland between 1975 and 1994," *Heart* 81, no. 4 (April 1999):
380–86, https://doi.org/10.1136/hrt.81.4.380; D. S. Jones and J. A. Greene, "The
Decline and Rise of Coronary Heart Disease: Understanding Public Health Catastro-
phism," *American Journal of Public Health* 103, no. 7 (July 2013): 1207–18, https://
doi.org/10.2105/AJPH.2013.301226; Schneider, *Invention of Surgery*; K. L. Syme
and E. H. Hagen, "Mental Health Is Biological Health: Why Tackling 'Diseases of
the Mind' Is an Imperative for Biological Anthropology in the 21st Century," *American Journal of Physical Anthropology* 171, suppl. 70 (May 2020): 87–117, https://doi
.org/10.1002/ajpa.23965.

   57. T. Andrasfay and N. Goldman, "Reductions in 2020 US Life Expectancy
Due to COVID-19 and the Disproportionate Impact on Black and Latino Popula-
tions," *Proceedings of the National Academy of Sciences* 118, no. 5 (January 14, 2021):
e2014746118, https://doi.org/10.1073/pnas.2014746118; E. Arias, K. D. Kochanek,
J. Xu, and B. Tejade-Vera, "Provisional Life Expectancy Estimates for 2022," *Vital
Statistics Surveillance Report*, no. 31 (November 2023), https://www.cdc.gov/nchs
/data/vsrr/vsrr031.pdf; K. M. Harris, S. H. Woolf, and D. J. Gaskin, "High and Rising
Working-Age Mortality in the US: A Report from the National Academies of Sciences,
Engineering, and Medicine," *JAMA* 325, no. 20 (May 25, 2021): 2045–46, https://
doi.org/10.1001/jama.2021.4073.

   58. Nuland, *Doctors*.

   59. Friedman and Friedland, *Medicine's 10 Greatest Discoveries*.

   60. Porter, "Medical Science."

   61. A. Flexner, *Medical Education in the United States and Canada: A Report to the Carnegie Foundation for the Advancement of Teaching* (New York: Carnegie Foundation, 1910).

   62. Starr, *Social Transformation of American Medicine*.

   63. Bradley and Tayor, *American Health Care Paradox*; E. J. Emanuel, *Prescription for
the Future: The Twelve Transformational Practices of Highly Effective Medical Organizations* (New York: PublicAffairs, 2017); Porter, "Medical Science"; C. E. Rosenberg, *The
Care of Strangers: The Rise of America's Hospital System* (New York: Basic Books, 1987).

   64. Porter, "Medical Science."

   65. Association of American Medical Colleges, *Basic Science, Foundational Knowledge*;
H. Leigh, R. Mallios, and D. Stewart, "Teaching Psychiatry in Primary Care Residen-
cies: Do Training Directors of Primary Care and Psychiatry See Eye to Eye?" *Academic
Psychiatry* 32, no. 6 (November–December 2008): 504–9, https://doi.org/10.1176
/appi.ap.32.6.504; H. Leigh, D. Stewart, and R. Mallios, "Mental Health and Psychiatry
Training in Primary Care Residency Programs: Part I: Who Teaches, Where, When and

How Satisfied?" *General Hospital Psychiatry* 28, no. 3 (May–June 2006): 189–94, https://doi.org/10.1016/j.genhosppsych.2005.10.003.

66. S. Browne and M. Burton, *The History of Psychiatry: Important Figures and Developments* (Scotts Valley, CA: CreateSpace Independent Publishing Platform, 2015); K. S. Kendler, K. Tabb, and J. Wright, "The Emergence of Psychiatry: 1650–1850," *American Journal of Psychiatry* 179, no. 5 (May 2022): 329–335, https://doi.org/10.1176/appi.ajp.21060614; Porter, *Greatest Benefit to Mankind*; R. Porter, "Mental Illness," in *Cambridge History of Medicine*, ed. R. Porter, 238–59 (Cambridge, UK: Cambridge University Press, 2011).

67. Browne and Burton, *History of Psychiatry*.

68. Browne and Burton, *History of Psychiatry*; Porter, *Greatest Benefit to Mankind*; Porter, "Mental Illness."

69. Browne and Burton, *History of Psychiatry*; Kendler, Tabb, and Wright, "Emergence of Psychiatry"; Porter, *Greatest Benefit to Mankind*.

70. Browne and Burton, *History of Psychiatry*; Porter, *Greatest Benefit to Mankind*.

71. Browne and Burton, *History of Psychiatry*; Kendler, Tabb, and Wright, "Emergence of Psychiatry"; Porter, *Greatest Benefit to Mankind*; Porter, "Mental Illness."

72. Browne and Burton, *History of Psychiatry*; A. Harrington, *Mind Fixers: Psychiatry's Troubled Search for the Biology of Mental Illness* (New York: W. W. Norton, 2019); Porter, *Greatest Benefit to Mankind*.

73. E. R. Kandel, *The Age of Insight: The Quest to Understand the Unconscious in Art, Mind, and Brain: From Vienna 1900 to the Present* (New York: Random House, 2012).

74. J. L. Levenson, *Textbook of Psychosomatic Medicine* (Washington, DC: American Psychiatric Association, 2005).

75. American Psychiatric Association, *Diagnostic and Statistical Manual of Mental Disorders: DSM-5*, 5th ed. (Washington, DC: American Psychiatric Association, 2013); R. C. Smith, D. D'Mello, G. G. Osborn, L. Freilich, F. C. Dwamena, and H. Laird-Fick, *Essentials of Psychiatry in Primary Care: Behavioral Health in the Medical Setting* (New York: McGraw Hill Education, 2019).

76. Browne and Burton, *History of Psychiatry*; C. Gardner and A. Kleinman, "Medicine and the Mind: The Consequences of Psychiatry's Identity Crisis," *New England Journal of Medicine* 381, no. 18 (October 31, 2019): 1697–99, https://doi.org/10.1056/NEJMp1910603; Harrington, *Mind Fixers*; A. Kleinman, "Rebalancing Academic Psychiatry: Why It Needs to Happen—and Soon," *British Journal of Psychiatry* 201, no. 6 (December 2012): 421–22, https://doi.org/10.1192/bjp.bp.112.118695; A. Kleinman, *Rethinking Psychiatry: From Cultural Category to Personal Experience* (New York: Free Press, 1988); R. Porter, *Greatest Benefit to Mankind*.

77. Kandel, *Age of Insight*.

78. Browne and Burton, *History of Psychiatry*.

79. Harrington, *Mind Fixers*.

80. Browne and Burton, *History of Psychiatry*; Harrington, *Mind Fixers*.

81. Harrington, *Mind Fixers*; T. R. Insel, "Balancing Immediate Needs with Future Innovation," *Director's Blog* (blog), 2012; T. R. Insel, *Healing: Our Path from Mental Illness to Mental Health* (New York: Penguin Books, 2022); K. S. Kendler, "From Many

to One to Many—The Search for Causes of Psychiatric Illness," *JAMA Psychiatry* 76, no. 10 (October 1, 2019): 1085–91, https://doi.org/10.1001/jamapsychiatry.2019.1200.

82. P. Bracken, P. Thomas, S. Timimi, E. Asen, G. Behr, C. Beuster, S. Bhunnoo et al., "Psychiatry beyond the Current Paradigm," *British Journal of Psychiatry* 201, no. 6 (December 2012): 430–34, https://doi.org/10.1192/bjp.bp.112.109447; Kendler, "From Many to One"; E. H. Rubin and C. F. Zorumski, "Perspective: Upcoming Paradigm Shifts for Psychiatry in Clinical Care, Research, and Education," *Academic Medicine* 87, no. 3 (March 2012): 261–65, https://doi.org/10.1097/ACM.0b013e3182441697.

83. J. R. Kriel, "Removing Medicine's Cartesian Mask: The Problem of Humanizing Medical Education: Part I," *Journal of Biblical Ethics in Medicine* 3, no. 2 (1989): 18–22, https://bmei.org/removing-medicines-cartesian-mask-the-problem-of-humanizing-med ical-education-part-i/.

84. Kriel, "Removing Medicine's Cartesian Mask"; Mehta, "Mind-Body Dualism"; G. Watts, "Looking to the Future," in *Cambridge History of Medicine*, ed. R. Porter, 298–329 (Cambridge, UK: Cambridge University Press, 2011).

85. S. Tomaselli, "The First Person: Descartes, Locke and Mind-Body Dualism," *History of Science* 22, pt. 2 (1984): 185–205, https://doi.org/10.1177/007327538402200203.

86. Watts, "Looking to the Future."

87. Brown, "Cartesian Dualism and Psychosomatics"; T. S. Kuhn, *The Structure of Scientific Revolutions* (Chicago: University of Chicago Press, 1962); Mehta, "Mind-Body Dualism."

88. Kuhn, *Structure of Scientific Revolutions*.

89. C. H. Hennekens and J. E. Buring, *Epidemiology in Medicine*, ed. S. L. Mayrent (Boston: Little, Brown, 1987); J. Jaccard and J. Jacoby, *Theory Construction and Model-Building Skills: A Practical Guide for Social Scientists* (New York: Guilford Press, 2010); D. Miller (ed.), *Popper Selections* (Princeton, NJ: Princeton University Press, 1984); K. R. Popper, *The Myth of the Framework: In Defence of Science and Rationality*, ed. M. A. Notturno (New York: Routledge, 1994); D. L. Sackett, R. B. Haynes, G. H. Guyaatt, and P. Tugwell, *Clinical Epidemiology: A Basic Science for Clinical Medicine*, 2nd ed. (Boston: Little, Brown, 1991); B. Spilker, *Guide to Clinical Trials* (Philadelphia: Lippincott, 1996); B. Spilker, introduction to *Quality of Life Assessments in Clinical Trials*, ed. B. Spilker, 3–9 (New York: Raven Press, 1990).

90. R. C. Smith, F. C. Dwamena, M. Grover, J. Coffey, and R. M. Frankel, "Behaviorally Defined Patient-Centered Communication—A Narrative Review of the Literature," *Journal of General Internal Medicine* 26, no. 2 (February 2011): 185–91, https://doi.org/10.1007/s11606-010-1496-5.

91. Brown, "Cartesian Dualism and Psychosomatics"; Capra and Luisi, *Systems View of Life*; Kriel, "Removing Medicine's Cartesian Mask."

92. Kuhn, *Structure of Scientific Revolutions*.

93. P. Sterling, *What Is Health? Allostasis and the Evolution of Human Design* (Cambridge, MA: MIT Press, 2020).

94. Capra and Luisi, *Systems View of Life*.

95. Capra and Luisi, *Systems View of Life*.

Chapter 6

1. F. Capra and P. Luisi, *The Systems View of Life: A Unifying Vision* (Cambridge, UK: Cambridge University Press, 2014).

2. S. Camazine, J.-L. Deneubourg, N. R. Franks, J. Sneyd, G. Theraulaz, and E. Bonabeau, *Self-Organization in Biological Systems* (Princeton, NJ: Princeton University Press, 2001); Capra and Luisi, *Systems View of Life*.

3. P. A. Weiss, *The Science of Life: The Living System—A System for Living* (Mount Kisco, NY: Futura, 1973).

4. J. Donne and W. Blake, *The Complete Poetry and Selected Prose of John Donne and the Complete Poetry of William Blake* (New York: Modern Library, 1941).

5. Capra and Luisi, *Systems View of Life*; Weiss, *Science of Life*.

6. Capra and Luisi, *Systems View of Life*; Weiss, *Science of Life*.

7. Capra and Luisi, *Systems View of Life*.

8. J. Levin, *A Madman Dreams of Turing Machines* (New York: Alfred A. Knopf, 2006); R. Schwarzlose, *Brainscapes: The Warped, Wondrous Maps Written in Your Brain—And How They Guide You* (Boston: Houghton Mifflin Harcourt, 2021).

9. Capra and Luisi, *Systems View of Life*; Levin, *Madman Dreams of Turing Machines*.

10. Capra and Luisi, *Systems View of Life*.

11. Capra and Luisi, *Systems View of Life*.

12. G. Bateson, *Mind and Nature: A Necessary Unity* (New York: Dutton, 1979); G. Bateson, *Steps to an Ecology of Mind: A Revolutionary Approach to Man's Understanding of Himself* (New York: Ballantine Books, 1972).

13. Capra and Luisi, *Systems View of Life*.

14. Capra and Luisi, *Systems View of Life*.

15. A. Koestler, "Beyond Atomism and Holism: The Concept of the Holon," in *Beyond Reductionism: New Perspectives in the Life Sciences*, ed. A. Koestler and J. R. Smythies, 192–232 (Boston: Beacon Press, 1969); L. von Bertalanffy, "Chance or Law," in *Beyond Reductionism: New Perspectives in the Life Sciences*, ed. A. Koestler and J. R. Smythies, 56–84 (Boston: Beacon Press, 1969); L. von Bertalanffy, *General System Theory: Foundations, Development, Application*, rev. ed. (New York: George Braziller, 1968); Weiss, *Science of Life*.

16. K. E. Boulding, "General Systems Theory—The Skeleton of Science," *Management Science* 2, no. 3 (April 1956): 197–208, https://www.jstor.org/stable/2627132; H. Brody, "The Systems View of Man: Implications for Medicine, Science, and Ethics," *Perspectives in Biology and Medicine* 17, no. 1 (Autumn 1973): 71–92, https://doi.org/10.1353/pbm.1973.0007; Weiss, *Science of Life*.

17. Camazine et al., *Self-Organization in Biological Systems*; L. Foss and K. Rothenberg, *The Second Medical Revolution: From Biomedicine to Infomedicine* (Boston: Shambhala, 1987); P. R. McHugh and P. R. Slavney, *The Perspectives of Psychiatry* (Baltimore, MD: Johns Hopkins University Press, 1986); M. A. Schwartz and O. P. Wiggins, "Systems and the Structuring of Meaning: Contributions to a Biopsychosocial Medicine," *American Journal of Psychiatry* 143, no. 10 (October 1986): 1213–21, https://doi.org/10.1176/ajp.143.10.1213.

18. D. Bolton and G. Gillett, *The Biopsychosocial Model of Health and Disease: New Philosophical and Scientific Developments* (Cham, Switzerland: Springer International, 2019); E. J. Cassell, *Doctoring: The Nature of Primary Care Medicine* (New York: Oxford University Press, 1997); L. Wynne, "Systems Theory and the Biopsychosocial Approach," in *The Biopsychosocial Approach: Past, Present, and Future*, ed. R. M. Frankel, T. E. Quill, and S. McDaniel, 220–30 (Rochester, NY: University of Rochester Press, 2003).

19. R. Ader, "Psychoneuroimmunology: Basic Research in the Biopsychosocial Approach," in *The Biopsychosocial Approach: Past, Present, and Future*, ed. R. M. Frankel, T. E. Quill, and S. McDaniel, 93–108 (Rochester, NY: University of Rochester Press, 2003).

20. G. L. Engel, "The Clinical Application of the Biopsychosocial Model," *American Journal of Psychiatry* 137, no. 5 (May 1980): 535–44, https://doi.org/10.1176/ajp.137.5.535; G. L. Engel, "The Need for a New Medical Model: A Challenge for Biomedicine," *Science* 196, no. 4286 (April 8, 1977): 129–36, https://doi.org/10.1126/science.847460; R. C. Smith, A. H. Fortin VI, F. Dwamena, and R. M. Frankel, "An Evidence-Based Patient-Centered Method Makes the Biopsychosocial Model Scientific," *Patient Education and Counseling* 91, no. 3 (June 2013): 265–70, https://doi.org/10.1016/j.pec.2012.12.010; R. C. Smith, "Making the Biopsychosocial Model More Scientific—Its General and Specific Models," *Social Science and Medicine* 272 (March 2021): 113568, https://doi.org/10.1016/j.socscimed.2020.113568.

21. J. Cohen and S. B. Clark, *John Romano and George Engel: Their Lives and Work* (Rochester, NY: Meliora Press, University of Rochester Press, 2010).

22. T. Brown, "George Engel and Rochester's Biopsychosocial Tradition: Historical and Developmental Perspectives," in *The Biopsychosocial Approach: Past, Present, and Future*, ed. R. M. Frankel, T. E. Quill, and S. McDaniel, 199–219 (Rochester, NY: University of Rochester Press, 2003).

23. Smith, Fortin et al., "Evidence-Based Patient-Centered Method"; Smith, "Making the Biopsychosocial Model."

24. G. L. Engel, foreword, in *The Second Medical Revolution: From Biomedicine to Infomedicine*, ed. L. Foss and K. Rothenberg, vii–ix (Boston: Shambhala, 1987); Foss and Rothenberg, *Second Medical Revolution*; O. Freudenreich, N. Kontos, and J. Querques, "The Muddles of Medicine: A Practical, Clinical Addendum to the Biopsychosocial Model," *Psychosomatics* 51, no. 5 (September–October 2010): 365–69, https://doi.org/10.1176/appi.psy.51.5.365; S. N. Ghaemi, "The Rise and Fall of the Biopsychosocial Model," *British Journal of Psychiatry* 195, no. 1 (July 2009): 3–4, https://doi.org/10.1192/bjp.bp.109.063859; J. Herman, "The Need for a Transitional Model: A Challenge for Biopsychosocial Medicine?" *Families, Systems, and Health* 23, no. 4 Winter 2005): 372–76, https://doi.org/10.1037/1091-7527.23.4.372; N. McLaren, "A Critical Review of the Biopsychosocial Model," *Australian and New Zealand Journal of Psychiatry* 32, no. 1 (February 1998): 86–92, discussion 93–96, https://doi.org/10.3109/00048679809062712; J. Z. Sadler and Y. F. Hulgus, "Knowing, Valuing, Acting: Clues to Revising the Biopsychosocial Model," *Comprehensive Psychiatry* 31, no. 3 (May–June 1990): 185–95, https://doi.org/10.1016/0010-440x(90)90001-9; M. A. Schwartz and O. Wiggins, "Science, Humanism, and the Nature of Medical Practice: A Phenomenological View," *Perspectives in Biology and Medicine* 28, no. 3 (Spring 1985): 331–66, https://doi.org/10.1353/pbm.1985.0008.

25. B. M. Korsch, "Current Issues in Communication Research," *Health Communications* 1, no. 1 (1989): 5–9, https://doi.org/10.1207/s15327027hc0101_1; B. M. Korsch, E. K. Gozzi, and V. Francis, "Gaps in Doctor-Patient Communication: 1. Doctor-Patient Interaction and Patient Satisfaction," *Pediatrics* 42, no. 5 (November 1968): 855–71, https://pubmed.ncbi.nlm.nih.gov/5685370/; B. M. Korsch and V. F. Negrete, "Doctor-Patient Communication," *Scientific American* 227, no. 2 (August 1972): 66–74, https://doi.org/10.1038/scientificamerican0872-66; W. L. Morgan Jr. and G. L. Engel, *The Clinical Approach to the Patient* (Philadelphia: Saunders, 1969).

26. Engel, foreword; Foss and Rothenberg, *Second Medical Revolution*; Freudenreich, Kontos, and Querques, "Muddles of Medicine"; Ghaemi, "Rise and Fall"; Herman, "Need for a Transitional Model"; McLaren, "Critical Review"; Sadler and Hulgus, "Knowing, Valuing, Acting"; Schwartz and Wiggins, "Science, Humanism."

27. Korsch, "Current Issues in Communication Research"; Korsch, Gozzi, and Francis, "Gaps in Doctor-Patient Communication"; Korsch and Negrete, "Doctor-Patient Communication"; Morgan and Engel, *Clinical Approach to the Patient*; C. R. Rogers, "The Characteristics of a Helping Relationship," *Personnel and Guidance Journal* 37, no. 1 (September 1958): 6–16, https://doi.org/10.1002/j.2164-4918.1958.tb01147.x; C. R. Rogers, *Client-Centered Therapy: Its Current Practice, Implications, and Theory* (Boston: Houghton Mifflin, 1951).

28. I. McWhinney, "The Need for a Transformed Clinical Method," in *Communicating with Medical Patients*, ed. M. Stewart and D. Roter, 25–42 (Newbury Park, CA: Sage, 1989).

29. J. Bird and S. A. Cohen-Cole, "The Three-Function Model of the Medical Interview: An Educational Device," in *Methods in Teaching Consultation-Liaison Psychiatry*, ed. M. S. Hale, 65–88 (Basel, Switzerland: Karger, 1990); S. A. Cole and J. Bird, *The Medical Interview: The Three Function Approach*, 3rd ed. (Philadelphia: Elsevier, Saunders, 2014); W. T. Branch, R. A. Arky, B. Woo, J. D. Stoeckle, D. B. Levy, and W. C. Taylor, "Teaching Medicine as a Human Experience: A Patient-Doctor Relationship Course for Faculty and First-Year Medical Students," *Annals of Internal Medicine* 114, no. 6 (March 15, 1991): 482–89, https://doi.org/10.7326/0003-4819-114-6-482; W. T. Branch and T. K. Malik, "Using 'Windows of Opportunities' in Brief Interviews to Understand Patients' Concerns," *JAMA* 269, no. 13 (April 7, 1993): 1667–68, https://doi.org/10.1001/jama.1993.03500130081036; J. Brown, "Perspective: Clinical Communication Education in the United Kingdom: Some Fresh Insights," *Academic Medicine* 87, no. 8 (August 2012): 1101–4, https://doi.org/10.1097/ACM.0b013e31825ccbb4; Cassell, *Doctoring*; E. J. Cassell, *Talking with Patients*, vol. 1: *The Theory of Doctor-Patient Communication* (Cambridge, MA: MIT Press, 1985); D. L. Duffy, D. Hammerman, and M. A. Cohen, "Communication Skills of House Officers: A Study in a Medical Clinic," *Annals of Internal Medicine* 93, no. 2 (August 1, 1980): 354–57, https://doi.org/10.7326/0003-4819-93-2-354; A. Lazare, S. M. Putnam, and M. Lipkin Jr., "Three Functions of the Medical Interview," in *The Medical Interview: Clinical Care, Education, and Research*, ed. M. Lipkin Jr., S. M. Putnam, and A. Lazare, 3–19 (New York: Springer-Verlag, 1995); M. Lipkin Jr., T. E. Quill, and R. J. Napodano, "The Medical Interview: A Core Curriculum for Residencies in Internal Medicine," *Annals of Internal Medicine* 100, no. 2 (February 1984): 277–84, https://doi.org/10.7326/0003

-4819-100-2-277; P. Maguire, S. Fairbairn, and C. Fletcher, "Consultation Skills of Young Doctors: I—Benefits of Feedback Training in Interviewing as Students Persist," *British Medical Journal* 292, no. 6535 (June 14, 1986): 1573–76, https://doi .org/10.1136/bmj.292.6535.1573; P. Maguire, P. Roe, D. Goldberg, S. Jones, C. Hyde, and T. O'Dowd, "The Value of Feedback in Teaching Interviewing Skills to Medical Students," *Psychological Medicine* 8, no. 4 (November 1978): 695–704, https://doi .org/10.1017/s0033291700018894; D. H. Novack, "Therapeutic Aspects of the Clinical Encounter," *Journal of General Internal Medicine* 2, no. 5 (September–October 1987): 346–55, https://doi.org/10.1007/BF02596174; F. W. Platt and J. C. McMath, "Clinical Hypocompetence: The Interview," *Annals of Internal Medicine* 91, no. 6 (December 1979): 898–902, https://doi.org/10.7326/0003-4819-91-6-898; S. M. Putnam, W. B. Stiles, M. C. Jacob, and S. A. James, "Teaching the Medical Interview: An Intervention Study," *Journal of General Internal Medicine* 3, no. 1 (January–February 1988): 38–47, https://doi.org/10.1007/BF02595755; T. E. Quill, "Partnerships in Patient Care: A Contractual Approach," *Annals of Internal Medicine* 98, no. 2 (February 1983): 228–34, https://doi.org/10.7326/0003-4819-98-2-228; T. E. Quill, "Recognizing and Adjusting to Barriers in Doctor-Patient Communication," *Annals of Internal Medicine* 111, no. 1 (July 1, 1989): 51–57, https://doi.org/10.7326/0003-4819-111-1-51; J. Silverman, S. Kurtz, and J. Draper, *Skills for Communicating with Patients*, 3rd ed. (London: Radcliffe, 2013); J. D. Stoeckle and J. A. Billings, "A History of History-Taking: The Medical Interview," *Journal of General Internal Medicine* 2, no. 2 (March–April 1987): 119–27, https://doi.org/10.1007/BF02596310; B. Stoffelmayr, R. B. Hoppe, and N. Weber, "Facilitating Patient Participation: The Doctor-Patient Encounter," *Primary Care* 16, no. 1 (March 1989): 265–78, https://doi.org/10.1016/S0095-4543(21)01321 -X; A. L. Suchman, K. Markakis, H. B. Beckman, and R. Frankel, "A Model of Empathic Communication in the Medical Interview," *JAMA* 277, no. 8 (February 26, 1997): 678–82, https://doi.org/10.1001/jama.1997.03540320082047; A. L. Suchman and D. A. Matthews, "What Makes the Patient-Doctor Relationship Therapeutic? Exploring the Connexional Dimension of Medical Care," *Annals of Internal Medicine* 108, no. 1 (January 1988): 125–30, https://doi.org/10.7326/0003-4819-108-1-125; P. R. Williamson, R. C. Smith, D. E. Kern, M. Lipkin Jr., L. R. Barker, R. B. Hoppe, and J. Florek, "The Medical Interview and Psychosocial Aspects of Medicine: Block Curricula for Residents," *Journal of General Internal Medicine* 7, no. 2 (March–April 1992): 235–42, https://doi.org/10.1007/BF02598023.

30. H. B. Beckman and R. M. Frankel, "The Effect of Physician Behavior on the Collection of Data," *Annals of Internal Medicine* 101, no. 5 (November 1, 1984): 692–96, https://doi.org/10.7326/0003-4819-101-5-692; J. Bensing, S. van Dulmen, and K. Tates, "Communication in Context: New Directions in Communication Research," *Patient Education and Counseling* 50, no. 1 (May 2003): 27–32, https://doi .org/10.1016/s0738-3991(03)00076-4; Brody, "Systems View of Man"; J. B. Brown, M. Boles, J. P. Mullooly, and W. Levinson, "Effect of Clinician Communication Skills Training on Patient Satisfaction: A Randomized, Controlled Trial," *Annals of Internal Medicine* 131, no. 11 (December 7, 1999): 822–29, https://doi.org/10.7326/0003 -4819-131-11-199912070-00004; J. G. Carroll and J. Monroe, "Teaching Medical Interviewing: A Critique of Educational Research and Practice," *Journal of Medical Edu-

cation 54, no. 6 (June 1979): 498–500, https://journals.lww.com/academicmedicine/ab stract/1979/06000/teaching_medical_interviewing__a_critique_of.9.aspx; D. J. Cegala and S. L. Broz, "Physician Communication Skills Training: A Review of Theoretical Backgrounds, Objectives and Skills," *Medical Education* 36, no. 11 (November 2002): 1004–16, https://doi.org/10.1046/j.1365-2923.2002.01331.x; A. Cox, D. Holbrook, and M. Rutter, "Psychiatric Interviewing Techniques VI: Experimental Study: Eliciting Feelings," *British Journal of Psychiatry* 139, no. 2 (August 1981): 144–52, https://doi .org/10.1192/bjp.139.2.144; A. Cox, M. Rutter, and D. Holbrook, "Psychiatric Interviewing Techniques: A Second Experimental Study: Eliciting Feelings," *British Journal of Psychiatry* 152, no. 1 (January 1988): 64–72, https://doi.org/10.1192/bjp.152.1.64; A. Cox, M. Rutter, and D. Holbrook, "Psychiatric Interviewing Techniques V: Experimental Study: Eliciting Factual Information," *British Journal of Psychiatry* 139, no. 1 (July 1981): 29–37, https://doi.org/10.1192/bjp.139.1.29; L. Del Piccolo, H. de Haes, C. Heaven, J. Jansen, W. Verheul, J. Bensing, S. Bergvik et al., "Development of the Verona Coding Definitions of Emotional Sequences to Code Health Providers' Responses (VR-CoDES-P) to Patient Cues and Concerns," *Patient Education and Counseling* 82, no. 2 (February 2011): 149–55, https://doi.org/10.1016/j.pec.2010.02.024; L. Del Piccolo and A. Finset, "Assessment of Nonverbal Communication in Clinical Encounters: Many Methodological Approaches, but No Gold Standard," *Patient Education and Counseling* 86, no. 3 (March 2012): 279–80, https://doi.org/10.1016/S0738-3991(12)00057-2; F. D. Duffy, "Assessing Communication Skills of Internal Medicine Residents: A Perspective from the ABIM," presentation at the 27th annual meeting of the Association of Behavioral Sciences in Medical Education, October 19, 1997; R. M. Frankel, "Cracking the Code: Theory and Method in Clinical Communication Analysis," *Health Communication* 13, no. 1 (2001): 101–10, https://doi.org/10.1207/S15327027HC1301_09; K. Hopkinson, A. Cox, and M. Rutter, "Psychiatric Interviewing Techniques III: Naturalistic Study: Eliciting Feelings," *British Journal of Psychiatry* 138, no. 5 (May 1981): 406–15, https://doi.org/10.1192/bjp.138.5.406; T. S. Inui, "The Virtue of Qualitative and Quantitative Research," *Annals of Internal Medicine* 125, no. 9 (November 1, 1996): 770–71, https://doi.org/10.7326/0003-4819-125-9-199611010-00012; T. S. Inui and W. B. Carter, "Design Issues in Research of Doctor-Patient Communication," in *Communicating with Medical Patients*, ed. M. Stewart and D. Roter, 286 (Newbury Park, CA: Sage, 1989); T. S. Inui and W. B. Carter, "Problems and Prospects for Health Services Research on Provider-Patient Communication," *Medical Care* 23, no. 5 (May 1985): 521–38, https://doi.org/10.1097/00005650-198505000-00013; Korsch, "Current Issues in Communication Research"; G. Makoul, E. Krupat, and C.-H. Chang, "Measuring Patient Views of Physician Communication Skills: Development and Testing of the Communication Assessment Tool," *Patient Education and Counseling* 67, no. 3 (August 2007): 333–42, https://doi.org/10.1016/j.pec.2007.05.005; E. G. Mishler, *The Discourse of Medicine: Dialectics of Medical Interviews* (Norwood, NJ: Ablex, 1984); S. M. Putnam, W. B. Stiles, M. C. Jacob, and S. A. James, "Patient Exposition and Physician Explanation in Initial Medical Interviews and Outcomes of Clinic Visits," *Medical Care* 23, no. 1 (January 1985): 74–83, https://doi.org/10.1097/00005650-198501000 -00008; D. Roter, "Which Facets of Communication Have Strong Effects on Outcome: A Meta-Analysis," in *Communicating with Medical Patients*, ed. M. Stewart and

D. Roter, 183–96 (Newbury Park, CA: Sage, 1989); D. L. Roter, R. M. Frankel, J. A. Hall, and D. Sluyter, "The Expression of Emotion through Nonverbal Behavior in Medical Visits: Mechanisms and Outcomes," *Journal of General Internal Medicine* 21, suppl. 1 (January 2006): S28–34, https://doi.org/10.1111/j.1525-1497.2006.00306.x; D. Roter and S. Larson, "The Roter Interaction Analysis System (RIAS): Utility and Flexibility for Analysis of Medical Interactions," *Patient Education and Counseling* 46, no. 4 (April 2002): 243–51, https://doi.org/10.1016/s0738-3991(02)00012-5; R. L. Street Jr., "The Many 'Disguises' of Patient-Centered Communication: Problems of Conceptualization and Measurement," *Patient Education and Counseling* 100, no. 11 (November 2017): 2131–34, https://doi.org/10.1016/j.pec.2017.05.008; R. L. Street Jr., G. Makoul, N. K. Arora, and R. M. Epstein, "How Does Communication Heal? Pathways Linking Clinician-Patient Communication to Health Outcomes," *Patient Education and Counseling* 74, no. 3 (March 2009): 295–301, https://doi.org/10.1016/j.pec.2008.11.015; R. L. Street Jr. and K. M. Mazor, "Clinician-Patient Communication Measures: Drilling Down into Assumptions, Approaches, and Analyses," *Patient Education and Counseling* 100, no. 8 (August 2017): 1612–18, https://doi.org/10.1016/j.pec.2017.03.021; H. Waitzkin, "Doctor-Patient Communication: Clinical Implications of Social Scientific Research," *JAMA* 252, no. 17 (November 2, 1984): 2441–46, https://doi.org/10.1001/jama.252.17.2441; C. Zimmermann, L. Del Piccolo, J. Bensing, S. Bergvik, H. De Haes, H. Eide, I. Fletcher et al., "Coding Patient Emotional Cues and Concerns in Medical Consultations: The Verona Coding Definitions of Emotional Sequences (VR-CoDES)," *Patient Education and Counseling* 82, no. 2 (February 2011): 141–48, https://doi.org/10.1016/j.pec.2010.03.017.

31. R. C. Smith and R. B. Hoppe, "The Patient's Story: Integrating the Patient- and Physician-Centered Approaches to Interviewing," *Annals of Internal Medicine* 115, no. 6 (September 15, 1991): 470–77, https://doi.org/10.7326/0003-4819-115-6-470.

32. R. C. Smith, *The Patient's Story: Integrated Patient-Doctor Interviewing* (Boston: Little, Brown, 1996).

33. R. M. Frankel and T. S. Stein, *The Four Habits of Highly Effective Clinicians: A Practical Guide* (Menlo Park: Kaiser Permanente Northern California Region, 1996).

34. A. H. Fortin VI, F. C. Dwamena, R. M. Frankel, B. L. Lepisto, and R. C. Smith, *Smith's Patient-Centered Interviewing: An Evidence-Based Method*, 4th ed. (New York: McGraw-Hill Education, 2018).

35. B. F. Jensen, P. Gulbrandsen, F. A. Dahl, E. Krupat, R. M. Frankel, and A. Finset, "Effectiveness of a Short Course in Clinical Communication Skills for Hospital Doctors: Results of a Crossover Randomized Controlled Trial (ISRCTN22153332)," *Patient Education and Counseling* 84, no. 2 (August 2011): 163–69, https://doi.org/10.1016/j.pec.2010.08.028; R. C. Smith, H. Laird-Fick, F. C. Dwamena, L. Freilich, B. Mavis, K. Grayson-Sneed, D. D'Mello, M. Spoolsstra, and D. Solomon, "Teaching Residents Mental Health Care," *Patient Education and Counseling* 101, no. 12 (December 2018): 2145–55, https://doi.org/10.1016/j.pec.2018.07.023; R. C. Smith, J. S. Lyles, J. Mettler, B. E. Stoffelmayr, L. F. Van Egeren, A. A. Marshall, J. C. Gardiner et al., "The Effectiveness of Intensive Training for Residents in Interviewing: A Randomized, Controlled Study," *Annals of Internal Medicine* 128, no. 2 (January 15, 1998): 118–26, https://doi.org/10.7326/0003-4819-128-2-199801150-00008.

36. R. C. Smith, J. C. Gardiner, Z. Luo, S. Schooley, L. Lamerato, and K. Rost, "Primary Care Physicians Treat Somatization," *Journal of General Internal Medicine* 24, no. 7 (July 2009): 829–32, https://doi.org/10.1007/s11606-009-0992-y; R. C. Smith, J. S. Lyles, J. C. Gardiner, C. Sirbu, A. Hodges, C. Collins, F. C. Dwamena et al., "Primary Care Clinicians Treat Patients with Medically Unexplained Symptoms: A Randomized Controlled Trial," *Journal of General Internal Medicine* 21, no. 7 (July 2006): 671–77, https://doi.org/10.1111/j.1525-1497.2006.00460.x.

37. D. L. Sackett, W. S. Richardson, W. Rosenberg, and R. B. Haynes, *Evidence-Based Medicine: How to Practice and Teach EBM* (New York: Churchill Livingstone, 1997).

38. Smith, "Making the Biopsychosocial Model"; Smith, Fortin et al., "Evidence-Based Patient-Centered Method."

39. Bolton and Gillett, *Biopsychosocial Model of Health*.

40. Fortin et al., *Smith's Patient-Centered Interviewing*; R. C. Smith, D. D'Mello, G. G. Osborn, L. Freilich, F. C. Dwamena, and H. Laird-Fick, *Essentials of Psychiatry in Primary Care: Behavioral Health in the Medical Setting* (New York: McGraw-Hill Education, 2019).

41. Rogers, *Client-Centered Therapy*.

42. R. C. Smith, "How to Effectively Communicate with Others: Empathic Skills Pave the Way for Successful Communication," *Psychology Today*, October 2, 2021, https://www.psychologytoday.com/us/blog/patient-zero/202110/how-effectively-communicate-others.

43. L. F. Barrett, *How Emotions Are Made: The Secret Life of the Brain* (Boston: Houghton Mifflin Harcourt, 2017); R. Buck, *Emotion: A Biosocial Synthesis* (New York: Cambridge University Press, 2014); A. D. Craig, "Significance of the Insula for the Evolution of Human Awareness of Feelings from the Body," *Annals of the New York Academy of the Sciences* 1225, no. 1 (April 2011): 72–82, https://doi.org/10.1111/j.1749-6632.2011.05990.x; A. R. Damasio, *The Feeling of What Happens: Body and Emotion in the Making of Consciousness* (New York: Harcourt Brace, 1999); J. LeDoux, "The Power of Emotions," in *States of Mind: New Discoveries about How Our Brains Make Us Who We Are*, ed. R. Conlan, 123–49 (New York: John Wiley, 1999); R. M. Nesse, *Good Reasons for Bad Feelings: Insights from the Frontier of Evolutionary Psychiatry* (New York: Dutton, 2019); E. F. Pace-Schott, M. C. Amole, T. Aue, M. Balconi, L. M. Bylsma, H. Critchley, H. A. Demaree et al., "Physiological Feelings," *Neuroscience and Biobehavioral Reviews* 103 (August 2019): 267–304, https://doi.org/10.1016/j.neubiorev.2019.05.002; J. Panksepp, "Neurologizing the Psychology of Affects: How Appraisal-Based Constructivism and Basic Emotion Theory Can Coexist," *Perspectives on Psychological Science* 2, no. 3 (September 2007): 281–96, https://doi.org/10.1111/j.1745-6916.2007.00045.x; B. A. van der Kolk, *The Body Keeps the Score: Brain, Mind, and Body in the Healing of Trauma* (New York: Penguin Books, 2014).

44. M. A. Stewart, "Effective Physician-Patient Communication and Health Outcomes: A Review," *Canadian Medical Association Journal* 152, no. 9 (May 1, 1995): 1423–33, https://pubmed.ncbi.nlm.nih.gov/7728691/.

45. M. Stewart, J. B. Brown, A. Donner, I. R. McWhinney, J. Oates, W. W. Weston, and J. Jordan, "The Impact of Patient-Centered Care on Outcomes," *Journal*

of Family Practice 49, no. 9 (September 2000): 796–804, https://pubmed.ncbi.nlm.nih
.gov/11032203/.

46. F. Dwamena, M. Holmes-Rovner, C. M. Gaulden, S. Jorgenson, G. Sadigh, A.
Sikorskii, S. Lewin, R. C. Smith, J. Coffey, and A. Olomu, "Interventions for Providers to Promote a Patient-Centred Approach in Clinical Consultations," *Cochrane Database of Systematic Reviews* 12, no. 12 (December 12, 2012): CD003267, https://doi
.org/10.1002/14651858.CD003267.pub2.

47. J. M. Kelley, G. Kraft-Todd, L. Schapira, J. Kossowsky, and H. Riess, "The
Influence of the Patient-Clinician Relationship on Healthcare Outcomes: A Systematic
Review and Meta-Analysis of Randomized Controlled Trials," *PLoS One* 9, no. 4 (April
9, 2014): e94207, https://doi.org/10.1371/journal.pone.0094207.

48. D. Spiegel, "Mind Matters in Cancer Survival," *Psycho-Oncology* 21, no. 6 (June
2012): 588–93, https://doi.org/10.1002/pon.3067.

49. D. S. Davydow and J. Unützer, "In Memoriam: Wayne Katon, MD (1950–
2015)," *General Hospital Psychiatry* 37, no. 3 (May–June 2015): 195–96, https://doi
.org/10.1016/j.genhosppsych.2015.03.013.

50. J. C. Huffman, S. K. Niazi, J. R. Rundell, M. Sharpe, and W. J. Katon, "Essential Articles on Collaborative Care Models for the Treatment of Psychiatric Disorders in
Medical Settings: A Publication by the Academy of Psychosomatic Medicine Research
and Evidence-Based Practice Committee," *Psychosomatics* 55, no. 2 (March–April 2014):
109–22, https://doi.org/10.1016/j.psym.2013.09.002; E. Woltmann, A. Grogan-
Kaylor, B. Perron, H. Georges, A. M. Kilbourne, and M. S. Bauer, "Comparative Effectiveness of Collaborative Chronic Care Models for Mental Health Conditions across
Primary, Specialty, and Behavioral Health Care Settings: Systematic Review and Meta-
Analysis," *American Journal of Psychiatry* 169, no. 8 (August 2012): 790–804, https://doi
.org/10.1176/appi.ajp.2012.11111616.

51. J. A. Hall, D. L. Roter, and N. R. Katz, "Meta-Analysis of Correlates of Provider
Behavior in Medical Encounters," *Medical Care* 26, no. 7 (July 1988): 657–75, https://
doi.org/10.1097/00005650-198807000-00002; E. Krupat, S. L. Rosenkranz, C. M.
Yeager, K. Barnard, S. M. Putnam, and T. S. Inui, "The Practice Orientations of Physicians and Patients: The Effect of Doctor-Patient Congruence on Satisfaction," *Patient
Education and Counseling* 39, no. 1 (January 2000): 49–59, https://doi.org/10.1016
/s0738-3991(99)00090-7; Z. A. Marcum, M. A. Sevick, and S. M. Handler, "Medication Nonadherence: A Diagnosable and Treatable Medical Condition," *JAMA* 309, no.
20 (May 22, 2013): 2105–6, https://doi.org/10.1001/jama.2013.4638.

52. W. Levinson, D. L. Roter, J. P. Mullooly, V. T. Dull, and R. M. Frankel,
"Physician-Patient Communication: The Relationship with Malpractice Claims among
Primary Care Physicians and Surgeons," *JAMA* 277, no. 7 (February 19, 1997): 553–59,
https://pubmed.ncbi.nlm.nih.gov/9032162/.

53. D. L. Roter, J. A. Hall, and N. R. Katz, "Relations between Physicians' Behaviors
and Analogue Patients' Satisfaction, Recall, and Impressions," *Medical Care* 25, no. 5
(May 1987): 437–51, https://doi.org/10.1097/00005650-198705000-00007.

54. Committee on Quality Health Care in America, Institute of Medicine, *Crossing
the Quality Chasm: A New Health System for the 21st Century* (Washington, DC: National
Academy Press, 2001).

55. J. L. Dienstag, "The Medical College Admission Test—Toward a New Balance," *New England Journal of Medicine* 365, no. 21 (November 24, 2011): 1955–57, https://doi.org/10.1056/NEJMp1110171; R. M. Kaplan, J. M. Satterfield, and R. S. Kington, "Building a Better Physician—The Case for the New MCAT," *New England Journal of Medicine* 366, no. 14 (April 5, 2012): 1265–68, https://doi.org/10.1056 /NEJMp1113274; D. G. Kirch, K. Mitchell, and C. Ast, "The New 2015 MCAT: Testing Competencies," *JAMA* 310, no. 21 (December 4, 2013): 2243–44, https://doi .org/10.1001/jama.2013.282093; R. M. Schwartzstein, G. C. Rosenfeld, R. Hilborn, S. H. Oyewole, and K. Mitchell, "Redesigning the MCAT Exam: Balancing Multiple Perspectives," *Academic Medicine* 88, no. 5 (May 2013): 560–67, https://doi.org/10.1097 /ACM.0b013e31828c4ae0.

56. Association of American Medical Colleges, *Core Entrustable Professional Activities for Entering Residency: Curriculum Developers' Guide* (Washington, DC: Association of American Medical Colleges, 2014); S. E. Weinberger, A. G. Pereira, W. F. Iobst, A. J. Mechaber, and M. S. Bronze, "Competency-Based Education and Training in Internal Medicine," *Annals of Internal Medicine* 153, no. 11 (December 7, 2010): 751–56, https://doi.org/10.7326/0003-4819-153-11-201012070-00009.

57. Association of American Medical Colleges, *Basic Science, Foundational Knowledge, and Pre-Clerkship Content: Average Number of Hours for Instruction/Assessment of Curriculum Subjects* (Washington, DC: Association of American Medical Colleges, 2012); R. J. Choi, R. M. Betancourt, M. P. DeMarco, and K. D. W. Bream, "Medical Student Exposure to Integrated Behavioral Health," *Academic Psychiatry* 43, no. 2 (April 2019): 191–95, https://doi.org/10.1007/s40596-018-0936-0; M. P. DeMarco, R. M. Betancourt, K. M. Everard, and K. D. W. Bream, "Identifying Prevalence and Characteristics of Behavioral Health Education in Family Medicine Clerkships: A CERA Study," *Family Medicine* 50, no. 1 (January 2018): 36–40, https://doi.org/10.22454 /FamMed.2018.994360.

58. H. Leigh, R. Mallios, and D. Stewart, "Teaching Psychiatry in Primary Care Residencies: Do Training Directors of Primary Care and Psychiatry See Eye to Eye?" *Academic Psychiatry* 32, no. 6 (November–December 2008): 504–9, https://doi .org/10.1176/appi.ap.32.6.504.

59. R. Porter, "Medical Science," in *Cambridge History of Medicine*, ed. R. Porter, 136–75 (Cambridge, UK: Cambridge University Press, 2011).

60. R. Pearl, *Uncaring: How the Culture of Medicine Kills Doctors and Patients* (New York: PublicAffairs, 2021).

61. Capra and Luisi, *Systems View of Life.*

62. Capra and Luisi, *Systems View of Life.*

63. J. R. Kriel, "Removing Medicine's Cartesian Mask: The Problem of Humanizing Medical Education: Part I," *Journal of Biblical Ethics in Medicine* 3, no. 2 (1989): 18–22, https://bmei.org/removing-medicines-cartesian-mask-the-problem-of-humanizing-med ical-education-part-i/.

64. Quoted in T. S. Kuhn, *The Structure of Scientific Revolutions* (Chicago: University of Chicago Press, 1962).

65. History World, "History of Communication," accessed June 16, 2024, http:// www.historyworld.net/wrldhis/PlainTextHistories.asp?ParagraphID=flt; R. Lucky, "The

Quickening of Science Communication," *Science* 289, no. 5477 (July 14, 2000): 259–64, https://doi.org/10.1126/science.289.5477.259.

66. History World, "History of Communication"; Lucky, "Quickening of Science Communication."

67. Lucky, "Quickening of Science Communication."

68. Lucky, "Quickening of Science Communication."

69. Capra and Luisi, *Systems View of Life*.

70. Kuhn, *Structure of Scientific Revolutions*.

71. B. Barber, "Resistance by Scientists to Scientific Discovery: This Source of resistance Has Yet to Be Given the Scrutiny Accorded Religious and Ideological Sources," *Science* 134, no. 3479 (September 1, 1961): 596–602, https://doi.org/10.1126/science.134.3479.596; M. Edelson, *Hypothesis and Evidence in Psychoanalysis* (Chicago: University of Chicago Press, 1984); Kuhn, *Structure of Scientific Revolutions*.

72. E. J. Emanuel, *Prescription for the Future: The Twelve Transformational Practices of Highly Effective Medical Organizations* (New York: PublicAffairs, 2017); Kuhn, *Structure of Scientific Revolutions*; Pearl, *Uncaring*.

73. P. Feyerabend, *Against Method*, 4th ed. (London: Verso, 2010).

74. R. Lewontin, *The Triple Helix: Gene, Organism, and Environment* (Cambridge, MA: Harvard University Press, 2000).

75. Kuhn, *Structure of Scientific Revolutions*.

76. Kuhn, *Structure of Scientific Revolutions*.

Chapter 7

1. Brainy Quote, "Albert Einstein Quotes," accessed June 16, 2024, https://www.brainyquote.com/authors/albert-einstein-quotes.

2. F. Capra and P. Luisi, *The Systems View of Life: A Unifying Vision* (Cambridge, UK: Cambridge University Press, 2014).

3. P. Wátzlawick, J. B. Bavelas, and D. D. Jackson, *Pragmatics of Human Communication: A Study of Interactional Patterns, Pathologies, and Paradoxes* (New York: W. W. Norton, 1967); P. Wátzlawick, J. H. Weakland, and R. Fisch, *Change: Principles of Problem Formation and Problem Resolution* (New York: W. W. Norton, 1974); R. Szostak, "Interdisciplinary Research as a Creative Design Process," in. *Creativity, Design Thinking and Interdisciplinarity*, ed. F. Darbellay, Z. Moody, and T. Lubart, 17–33 (New York: Springer, 2017).

4. J. C. Huffman, S. K. Niazi, J. R. Rundell, M. Sharpe, and W. J. Katon, "Essential Articles on Collaborative Care Models for the Treatment of Psychiatric Disorders in Medical Settings: A Publication by the Academy of Psychosomatic Medicine Research and Evidence-Based Practice Committee," *Psychosomatics* 55, no. 2 (March–April 2014): 109–22, https://doi.org/10.1016/j.psym.2013.09.002; T. R. Insel, *Healing: Our Path from Mental Illness to Mental Health* (New York: Penguin Books, 2022); R. Kathol, S. Melek, S. Sargent, L. Sacks, and K. K. Patel, "Non-Traditional Mental Health and Substance Use Disorder Services as a Core Part of Health in CINs and ACOs,"

in *Clinical Integration: Population Health and Accountable Care*, 3rd ed., ed. K. Yale, T. A. Raskauskas, J. Bohn, and C. Konschak, 380–425 (Virginia Beach, VA: Convergent, 2015); P. P. Ramanuj and H. A. Pincus, "Collaborative Care: Enough of the Why; What about the How?" *British Journal of Psychiatry* 215, no. 4 (October 2019): 1–4, https://doi.org/10.1192/bjp.2019.99; K. Rost, P. Nutting, J. Smith, J. C. Coyne, L. Cooper-Patrick, and L. Rubenstein, "The Role of Competing Demands in the Treatment Provided Primary Care Patients with Major Depression," *Archives of Family Medicine* 9, no. 2 (February 2000): 150–54, https://doi.org/10.1001/archfami.9.2.150; P. Roy-Byrne, "Collaborative Care at the Crossroads," *British Journal of Psychiatry* 203, no. 2 (August 2013): 86–87, https://doi.org/10.1192/bjp.bp.113.128728.

5. D. Epstein, *Range: Why Generalists Triumph in a Specialized World* (New York: Riverhead Books, 2019); P. Feyerabend, *Against Method*, 4th ed. (London: Verso, 2010).

6. T. R. Insel, "Roads Not Taken," *Director's Blog* (blog), 2012.

7. T. R. Insel, "Balancing Immediate Needs with Future Innovation," *Director's Blog* (blog), 2012; Insel, *Healing*; Insel, "Roads Not Taken"; T. R. Insel, "Translating Scientific Opportunity into Public Health Impact: A Strategic Plan for Research on Mental Illness," *Archives of General Psychiatry* 66, no. 2 (February 2009): 128–33, https://doi.org/10.1001/archgenpsychiatry.2008.540; A. Kleinman, "Rebalancing Academic Psychiatry: Why It Needs to Happen—and Soon," *British Journal of Psychiatry* 201, no. 6 (December 2012): 421–22, https://doi.org/10.1192/bjp.bp.112.118695; D. Mechanic, "More People than Ever Before Are Receiving Behavioral Health Care in the United States, but Gaps and Challenges Remain," *Health Affairs* 33, no. 8 (August 2014): 1416–24, https://doi.org/10.1377/hlthaff.2014.0504; R. N. Nesse, *Good Reasons for Bad Feelings: Insights from the Frontier of Evolutionary Psychiatry* (New York: Dutton, 2019).

8. G. H. Gibbons, C. E. Seidman, and E. J. Topol, "Conquering Atherosclerotic Cardiovascular Disease—50 Years of Progress," *New England Journal of Medicine* 384, no. 9 (March 4, 2021): 785–88, https://doi.org/10.1056/NEJMp2033115.

9. Nesse, *Good Reasons for Bad Feelings*; B. A. van der Kolk, *The Body Keeps the Score: Brain, Mind, and Body in the Healing of Trauma* (New York: Penguin Books, 2014).

10. Nesse, *Good Reasons for Bad Feelings*.

11. Szostak, "Interdisciplinary Research"; Wátzlawick, Bavelas, and Jackson, *Pragmatics of Human Communication*; Wátzlawick, Weakland, and Fisch, *Change*.

12. Wátzlawick, Weakland, and Fisch, *Change*.

13. Szostak, "Interdisciplinary Research"; Wátzlawick, Weakland, and Fisch, *Change*.

14. D. Goleman, *Emotional Intelligence* (New York: Bantam Books, 1995); J. J. Gross, "Emotion Regulation: Past, Present, Future," *Cognition and Emotion* 13, no. 5 (1999): 551–73, https://doi.org/10.1080/026999399379186; J. J. Gross and R. W. Levenson, "Emotional Suppression: Physiology, Self-Report, and Expressive Behavior," *Journal of Personality and Social Psychology* 64, no. 6 (June 1993): 970–86, https://doi.org/10.1037//0022-3514.64.6.970; M. C. Schlatter and L. D. Cameron, "Emotional Suppression Tendencies as Predictors of Symptoms, Mood, and Coping Appraisals during AC Chemotherapy for Breast Cancer Treatment," *Annals of Behavioral Medicine* 40, no. 1 (August 2010): 15–29, https://doi.org/10.1007/s12160-010-9204-6.

15. Wátzlawick, Weakland, and Fisch, *Change*.

16. G. W. Allport, *The Nature of Prejudice* (Garden City, NY: Doubleday, 1958).

17. J. Stuber, I. Meyer, and B. Link, "Stigma, Prejudice, Discrimination and Health," *Social Science and Medicine* 67, no. 3 (August 2008): 351–57, https://doi.org/10.1016/j.socscimed.2008.03.023; G. Thornicroft, D. Rose, A. Kassam, and N. Sartorius, "Stigma: Ignorance, Prejudice or Discrimination?" *British Journal of Psychiatry* 190, no. 3 (March 2007): 192–93, https://doi.org/10.1192/bjp.bp.106.025791.

18. N. D. Volkow, "Stigma and the Toll of Addiction," *New England Journal of Medicine* 382, no. 14 (April 2, 2020): 1289–90, https://doi.org/10.1056/NEJMp1917360.

19. Thornicroft et al., "Stigma."

20. Committee on the Science of Changing Behavioral Health Social Norms, *Ending Discrimination against People with Mental and Substance Use Disorders: The Evidence for Stigma Change* (Washington, DC: National Academies Press, 2016).

21. US Department of Health and Human Services, "US Surgeon General Issues Advisory on Youth Mental Health Crisis Further Exposed by COVID-19 Pandemic," Southeast ADA Center, December 14, 2021, https://adasoutheast.org/u-s-sur geon-general-issues-advisory-on-youth-mental-health-crisis-further-exposed-by-covid -19-pandemic/.

22. C.-H. Au, C. S.-M. Wong, C.-W. Law, M.-C. Wong, and K.-F. Chung, "Self-Stigma, Stigma Coping and Functioning in Remitted Bipolar Disorder," *General Hospital Psychiatry* 57 (March–April 2019): 7–12, https://doi.org/10.1016/j.genhosp psych.2018.12.007.

23. J. L. Givens, I. R. Katz, S. Bellamy, and W. C. Holmes, "Stigma and the Acceptability of Depression Treatments among African Americans and Whites," *Journal of General Internal Medicine* 22, no. 9 (September 2007): 1292–97, https://doi.org/10.1007 /s11606-007-0276-3.

24. R. L. Kravitz, D. A. Paterniti, R. M. Epstein, A. B. Rochlen, R. A. Bell, C. Cipri, E. Fernandez y Garcia, M. D. Feldman, and P. Duberstein, "Relational Barriers to Depression Help-Seeking in Primary Care," *Patient Education and Counseling* 82, no. 2 (February 2011): 207–13, https://doi.org/10.1016/j.pec.2010.05.007.

25. R. Horton, "Launching a New Movement for Mental Health," *Lancet* 370, no. 9590 (September 8, 2007): 806, https://doi.org/10.1016/S0140-6736(07)61243-4.

26. K. C. Soh, W. S. Lim, L. M. Cheang, and K. L. Chan, "Stigma towards Alcohol Use Disorder: Comparing Healthcare Workers with the General Population," *General Hospital Psychiatry* 58 (May–June 2019): 39–44, https://doi.org/10.1016/j.genhosp psych.2019.01.001.

27. S. Jilani, "Why So Many Doctors Treat Their Mental Health in Secret," *New York Times*, March 30, 2022, https://www.nytimes.com/2022/03/30/opinion/doctors -mental-health-stigma.html?searchResultPosition=1.

28. B. Maser, M. Danilewitz, E. Guérin, L. Findlay, and E. Frank, "Medical Student Psychological Distress and Mental Illness Relative to the General Population: A Canadian Cross-Sectional Survey," *Academic Medicine* 94, no. 11 (November 2019): 1781–91, https://doi.org/10.1097/ACM.0000000000002958; L. S. Rotenstein, M. A. Ramos, M. Torre, J. B. Segal, M. J. Peluso, C. Guille, S. Sen, and D. A. Mata, "Prevalence of Depression, Depressive Symptoms, and Suicidal Ideation among Medical Students: A Systematic Review and Meta-Analysis," *JAMA* 316, no. 21 (December 6, 2016): 2214–36, https://doi.org/10.1001/jama.2016.17324.

29. A. G. Greenwald, D. E. McGhee, and J. L. Schwartz, "Measuring Individual Differences in Implicit Cognition: The Implicit Association Test," *Journal of Personality and Social Psychology* 74, no. 6 (June 1998): 1464–80, https://doi.org/10.1037//0022 -3514.74.6.1464; Committee on the Science of Changing Behavioral Health Social Norms, *Ending Discrimination against People*; Thornicroft et al., "Stigma."

30. Committee on the Science of Changing Behavioral Health Social Norms, *Ending Discrimination against People*; G. Ivbijaro (ed.), *Companion to Primary Care Mental Health* (London: Wonca and Radcliffe, 2012); "A Decade for Psychiatric Disorders," *Nature* 463, no. 9 (January 7, 2010): 9, https://doi.org/10.1038/463009a; E. E. McGinty and C. L. Barry, "Stigma Reduction to Combat the Addiction Crisis—Developing an Evidence Base," *New England Journal of Medicine* 382, no. 14 (April 2, 2020): 1291–92, https://doi.org/10.1056/NEJMp2000227.

31. McGinty and Barry, "Stigma Reduction"; Committee on the Science of Changing Behavioral Health Social Norms, *Ending Discrimination against People*.

32. Thornicroft et al., "Stigma."

33. T. Ito, G. Urland, E. Willadsen-Jensen, and J. Correll, "The Social Neuroscience of Stereotyping and Prejudice: Using Event-Related Brain Potentials to Study Social Perception," in *Social Neuroscience: People Thinking about Thinking People*, ed. J. T. Cacioppo, P. S. Visser, and C. L. Pickett, 189–208 (Cambridge, MA: MIT Press, 2006).

34. J. T. Cacioppo, D. G. Amaral, J. J. Blanchard, J. L. Cameron, C. S. Carter, D. Crews, S. Fiske et al., "Social Neuroscience: Progress and Implications for Mental Health," *Perspectives on Psychological Science* 2, no. 2 (June 2007): 99–123, https://doi .org/10.1111/j.1745-6916.2007.00032.x; *Social Neuroscience and Behavior: From Basic to Clinical Science* (Washington, DC: National Institute of Mental Health, 2007); Goleman, *Emotional Intelligence*.

35. H. Benson, *The Relaxation Response* (New York: William Morrow, 1975); J. Kabat-Zinn, *Wherever You Go, There You Are: Mindfulness Meditation in Everyday Life* (New York: Hyperion, 1994); H. Stone and S. Stone, *Embracing Your Inner Critic: Turning Self-Criticism into a Creative Asset* (San Francisco: HarperSanFrancisco, 1993).

36. Capra and Luisi, *Systems View of Life*.

37. R. Porter, "Mental Illness," in *Cambridge History of Medicine*, ed. R. Porter, 238–59 (Cambridge, UK: Cambridge University Press, 2011).

38. Capra and Luisi, *Systems View of Life*.

39. Porter, "Mental Illness."

40. Porter, "Mental Illness."

41. O. W. Brawley and P. Goldberg, *How We Do Harm: A Doctor Breaks Ranks about Being Sick in America* (New York: St. Martin's Press, 2012); J. Geyman, "The Business Ethic vs. Service Ethic in US Health Care: Which Will Prevail?" *Pharos* (Winter 2022): 40–47, https://www.alphaomegaalpha.org/wp-content/uploads/2022/02 /p40-47_Ethics_Geyman__WIN22.pdf; M. Makary, *The Price We Pay: What Broke American Health Care—and How to Fix It* (New York: Bloomsbury, 2019); D. Mechanic, *From Advocacy to Allocation: The Evolving American Health Care System* (New York: Free Press, 1986); G. Moon and R. Gillespie, *Society and Health: An Introduction to Social Science for Health Professionals* London: Routledge, 1995); E. Rosenthal, *An American Sickness: How Healthcare Became Big Business and How You Can Take It Back*

(New York: Penguin Books, 2018); P. Starr, *The Social Transformation of American Medicine* (New York: Basic Books, 1982).

42. Starr, *Social Transformation of American Medicine*.

43. R. Pearl, *Uncaring: How the Culture of Medicine Kills Doctors and Patients* (New York: PublicAffairs, 2021).

44. M. Foucault, *The Birth of the Clinic: An Archeology of Medical Perception*, trans. A. M. S. Smith (New York: Vintage Books, 1973).

45. D. E. Hough, *Irrationality in Health Care: What Behavioral Economics Reveals about What We Do and Why* (Stanford, CA: Stanford University Press, 2013); C. E. Rosenberg, *The Care of Strangers: The Rise of America's Hospital System* (New York: Basic Books, 1987); Starr, *Social Transformation of American Medicine*.

46. Rosenthal, *American Sickness*; Starr, *Social Transformation of American Medicine*.

47. K. Armstrong and D. A. Asch, "Bridging Polarization in Medicine—From Biology to Social Causes," *New England Journal of Medicine* 382, no. 10 (March 5, 2020): 888–89, https://doi.org/10.1056/NEJMp1913051.

48. D. M. Berwick, "The Moral Determinants of Health," *JAMA* 324, no. 3 (July 21, 2020): 225–26, https://doi.org/10.1001/jama.2020.11129.

49. H. Arendt, *The Human Condition*, 2nd ed. (Chicago: University of Chicago Press, 2018).

50. E. H. Bradley and L. A. Tayor, *The American Health Care Paradox: Why Spending More Is Getting Us Less* (New York: PublicAffairs, 2013); R. Porter, "Medical Science," in *Cambridge History of Medicine*, ed. R. Porter, 136–75 (Cambridge, UK: Cambridge University Press, 2011); Rosenberg, *Care of Strangers*; Rosenthal, *American Sickness*; Starr, *Social Transformation of American Medicine*.

51. Starr, *Social Transformation of American Medicine*.

52. Rosenberg, *Care of Strangers*.

53. Rosenberg, *Care of Strangers*.

54. S. Brill, *America's Bitter Pill: Money, Politics, Backroom Deals, and the Fight to Fix Our Broken Healthcare System* (New York: Random House, 2015); Rosenthal, *American Sickness*; A. M. Sisko, S. P. Keehan, J. A. Poisal, G. A. Cuckler, S. D. Smith, A. J. Madison, K. E. Rennie, and J. C. Hardesty, "National Health Expenditure Projections, 2018–27: Economic and Demographic Trends Drive Spending and Enrollment Growth," *Health Affairs* 38, no. 3 (March 2019): 491–501, https://doi.org/10.1377/hlthaff.2018.05499.

55. Bradley and Tayor, *American Health Care Paradox*; Rosenthal, *American Sickness*.

56. Rosenthal, *American Sickness*.

57. Brill, *America's Bitter Pill*; Rosenthal, *American Sickness*.

58. R. Kluender, N. Mahoney, F. Wong, and W. Yin, "Medical Debt in the US, 2009–2020," *JAMA* 326, no. 3 (July 20, 2021): 250–56, https://doi.org/10.1001/jama.2021.8694.

59. Rosenthal, *American Sickness*.

60. Makary, *Price We Pay*.

61. Makary, *Price We Pay*; Rosenthal, *American Sickness*.

62. Rosenthal, *American Sickness*.

63. Geyman, "Business Ethic vs. Service Ethic."

64. Rosenthal, *American Sickness*.

65. Rosenthal, *American Sickness*.

66. Makary, *Price We Pay*.

67. Rosenthal, *American Sickness*.

68. D. M. Berwick, "Moral Choices for Today's Physician," *JAMA* 323, no. 17 (May 5, 2020): 1708–9, https://doi.org/10.1001/jama.2020.2984; Berwick, "Moral Determinants of Health"; A. Colby and W. Sullivan, "Formation of Professionalism and Purpose: Perspectives from the Preparation for the Professions Program," *University of St. Thomas Law Journal* 5, no. 2 (Winter 2008): 404–27, https://researchon line.stthomas.edu/esploro/outputs/journalArticle/Formation-of-Professionalism-and -Purpose-Perspectives/991015131240103691; A. Naess, *Ecology of Wisdom* (London: Penguin Classics, 2016).

69. D. M. Berwick, "*Salve Lucrum*: The Existential Threat of Greed in US Health Care," *JAMA* 329, no. 8 (February 28, 2023): 629–30, https://doi.org/10.1001 /jama.2023.0846; Brill, *America's Bitter Pill*; J. D. Bruch, V. Roy, and C. M. Grogan, "The Financialization of Health in the United States," *New England Journal of Medicine* 390, no. 2 (January 11, 2024): 178–82, https://doi.org/10.1056/NEJMms2308188; E. J. Emanuel, *Prescription for the Future: The Twelve Transformational Practices of Highly Effective Medical Organizations* (New York: PublicAffairs, 2017); Geyman, "Business Ethic vs. Service Ethic"; R. Pearl, *Mistreated: Why We Think We're Getting Good Health Care and Why We're Usually Wrong* (New York: PublicAffairs, 2017); Pearl, *Uncaring*; T. R. Reid, *The Healing of America: A Global Quest for Better, Cheaper, and Fairer Health Care* (New York: Penguin Books, 2009); Rosenthal, *American Sickness*.

70. Rosenthal, *American Sickness*.

71. A. Colby and W. Damon, *Some Do Care: Contemporary Lives of Moral Commitment* (New York: Free Press, 1992); Colby and Sullivan, "Formation of Professionalism"; Geyman, "Business Ethic vs. Service Ethic"; R. Nader, *Unsafe at Any Speed: The Designed-In Dangers of the American Automobile* (New York: Grossman, 1965).

72. Starr, *Social Transformation of American Medicine*.

73. Makary, *Price We Pay*.

74. Pearl, *Mistreated*.

75. S. Milgram, *Obedience to Authority: An Experimental View* (New York: Harper & Row, 1974); Pearl, *Mistreated*.

76. C. Romm, "Rethinking One of Psychology's Most Infamous Experiments," *Atlantic*, January 28, 2015, https://www.theatlantic.com/health/archive/2015/01/rethink-ing-one-of-psychologys-most-infamous-experiments/384913/; J. J. Van Bavel and D. J. Packer, *The Power of Us: Harnessing Our Shared Identities to Improve Performance, Increase Cooperation, and Promote Social Harmony* (New York: Little, Brown Spark, 2021).

77. Milgram, *Obedience to Authority*.

78. Milgram, *Obedience to Authority*.

79. Milgram, *Obedience to Authority*.

80. Milgram, *Obedience to Authority*.

81. Pearl, *Mistreated*.

82. Van Bavel and Packer, *Power of Us*.

83. Hough, *Irrationality in Health Care*; Pearl, *Mistreated*; Rosenthal, *American Sickness*.

84. Pearl, *Mistreated*.

Chapter 8

1. F. W. Walbank, "Alexander the Great: King of Macedonia," Britannica, updated April 30, 2024, https://www.britannica.com/biography/Alexander-the-Great.

2. D. M. Berwick, "The Moral Determinants of Health," *JAMA* 324, no. 3 (July 21, 2020): 225–26, https://doi.org/10.1001/jama.2020.11129.

3. D. M. Berwick, "Moral Choices for Today's Physician," *JAMA* 318, no. 21 (December 5, 2017): 2081–82, https://doi.org/10.1001/jama.2017.16254; Berwick, "Moral Determinants of Health."

4. W. Shakespeare, *The Complete Works of William Shakespeare* (San Diego: Canterbury Classics, 2014).

5. D. M. Berwick and J. A. Finkelstein, "Preparing Medical Students for the Continual Improvement of Health and Health Care: Abraham Flexner and the New 'Public Interest,'" *Academic Medicine* 85, suppl. 9 (September 2010): S56–65, https://doi.org/10.1097/ACM.0b013e3181ead779; M. Cooke, D. M. Irby, and B. C. O'Brien, *Educating Physicians: A Call for Reform of Medical School and Residency* (San Francisco: Jossey-Bass, 2010); M. Cooke, D. M. Irby, W. Sullivan, and K. M. Ludmerer, "American Medical Education 100 Years after the Flexner Report," *New England Journal of Medicine* 355, no. 13 (September 28, 2006): 1339–44, https://doi.org/10.1056/NEJMra055445; D. J. Doukas, L. B. McCullough, and S. Wear, "Re-visioning Flexner: Educating Physicians to Be Clinical Scientists and Humanists," *American Journal of Medicine* 123, no. 12 (December 2010): 1155–56, https://doi.org/10.1016/j.amjmed.2010.05.027; E. J. Emanuel, "Changing Premed Requirements and the Medical Curriculum," *JAMA* 296, no. 9 (September 6, 2006): 1128–31, https://doi.org/10.1001/jama.296.9.1128; J. Frenk, L. Chen, Z. A. Bhutta, J. Cohen, N. Crisp, T. Evans, H. Fineberg et al., "Health Professionals for a New Century: Transforming Education to Strengthen Health Systems in an Interdependent World," *Lancet* 376, no. 9756 (December 4, 2010): 1923–58, https://doi.org/10.1016/S0140-6736(10)61854-5; B. D. Hodges, "A *Tea-Steeping* or *i-Doc* Model for Medical Education?" *Academic Medicine* 85, suppl. 9 (September 2010): S34–44, https://doi.org/10.1097/ACM.0b013e3181f12f32; T. S. Inui, *A Flag in the Wind: Educating for Professionalism in Medicine* (Washington, DC: Association of American Medical Colleges, February 2003), https://med.fsu.edu/sites/default/files/userFiles/file/professinalism.pdf; K. M. Ludmerer, *Time to Heal: American Medical Education from the Turn of the Century to the Era of Managed Care* (Oxford, UK: Oxford University Press, 1999); S. E. Skochelak and S. J. Stack, "Creating the Medical Schools of the Future," *Academic Medicine* 92, no. 1 (January 2017): 16–19, https://doi.org/10.1097/ACM.0000000000001160; S. A. Wartman, "The Empirical Challenge of 21st-Century Medical Education," *Academic Medicine* 94, no. 10 (October

2019): 1412–15, https://doi.org/10.1097/ACM.0000000000002866; M. E. Whitcomb, "Commentary: Flexner Redux 2010: *Graduate* Medical Education in the United States," *Academic Medicine* 84, no. 11 (November 2009): 1476–78, https://doi.org/10.1097 /ACM.0b013e3181bb25db; M. E. Whitcomb, "Medical Education Reform: Is It Time for a Modern Flexner Report?" *Academic Medicine* 82, no. 1 (January 2007): 1–2, https://doi.org/10.1097/ACM.0b013e31802be06e.

6. R. Pearl, *Uncaring: How the Culture of Medicine Kills Doctors and Patients* (New York: PublicAffairs, 2021).

7. Brainy Quote, "Aldous Huxley Quotes," accessed June 17, 2024, https://www .brainyquote.com/authors/aldous-huxley-quotes.

8. Berwick, "Moral Determinants of Health."

9. O. W. Brawley and P. Goldberg, *How We Do Harm: A Doctor Breaks Ranks about Being Sick in America* (New York: St. Martin's Press, 2012); M. Makary, *The Price We Pay: What Broke American Health Care—and How to Fix It* (New York: Bloomsbury, 2019); R. Nader, *Unsafe at Any Speed: The Designed-In Dangers of the American Automobile* (New York: Grossman, 1965).

10. F. Capra and P. Luisi, *The Systems View of Life: A Unifying Vision* (Cambridge, UK: Cambridge University Press, 2014); P. Feyerabend, *Against Method*, 4th ed. (London: Verso, 2010); S. Johnson, *Extra Life: A Short History of Living Longer* (New York: Riverhead Books, 2021); T. S. Kuhn, *The Structure of Scientific Revolutions* (Chicago: University of Chicago Press, 1962); A. Naess, *Ecology of Wisdom* (London: Penguin Classics, 2016).

11. Johnson, *Extra Life*; Nader, *Unsafe at Any Speed*; R. Carson, *Silent Spring* (Boston: Houghton Mifflin, 1962).

12. Berwick, "Moral Determinants of Health."

13. R. Nader, *The Seventeen Solutions: Bold Ideas for Our American Future* (New York: Harper, 2012).

14. Berwick, "Moral Determinants of Health."

15. A. Colby and W. Sullivan, "Formation of Professionalism and Purpose: Perspectives from the Preparation for the Professions Program," *University of St. Thomas Law Journal* 5, no. 2 (Winter 2008): 404–27, https://researchonline.stthomas.edu /esploro/outputs/journalArticle/Formation-of-Professionalism-and-Purpose-Perspec tives/991015131240103691.

16. National Center for Health Statistics, "Anxiety and Depression," Centers for Disease Control and Prevention, reviewed June 14, 2024, https://www.cdc.gov/nchs /covid19/pulse/mental-health.htm; M. É. Czeisler, R. I. Lane, E. Petrosky, J. F. Wiley, A. Christensen, R. Njai, M. D. Weaver et al., "Mental Health, Substance Use, and Suicidal Ideation during the COVID-19 Pandemic—United States, June 24–30, 2020," *Morbidity and Mortality Weekly Report*, 69, no. 32 (August 14, 2020): 1049–57, https:// www.cdc.gov/mmwr/volumes/69/wr/pdfs/mm6932a1-H.pdf.

17. Czeisler et al., "Mental Health, Substance Use"; Colby and Sullivan, "Formation of Professionalism and Purpose"; N. Panchal, H. Saunders, R. Rudowitz, and C. Cox, "The Implications of COVID-19 for Mental Health and Substance Use," Kaiser Family Foundation, March 20, 2023, https://www.kff.org/coronavirus-covid-19/issue-brief/the -implications-of-covid-19-for-mental-health-and-substance-use/.

18. Quoted in Office of the Surgeon General, *Protecting Youth Mental Health: The US Surgeon General's Advisory* (Washington, DC: Department of Health and Human Services, 2021), https://www.hhs.gov/sites/default/files/surgeon-general-youth-mental -health-advisory.pdf.

19. R. Mishori, "The Social Determinants of Health? Time to Focus on the Political Determinants of Health!" *Medical Care* 57, no. 7 (July 2019): 491–93, https://doi .org/10.1097/MLR.0000000000001131.

20. J. Biden, "Remarks of President Joe Biden—State of the Union Address as Prepared for Delivery," White House, March 1, 2022, https://www.whitehouse.gov /briefing-room/speeches-remarks/2022/03/01/remarks-of-president-joe-biden-state-of -the-union-address-as-delivered/.

21. A. H. Krist, J. South-Paul, and M. Meisnere (eds.), *Achieving Whole Health: A New Approach for Veterans and the Nation* (Washington, DC: National Academies Press, 2023), http://nap.nationalacademies.org/26854.

22. Feyerabend, *Against Method.*

23. A. Flexner, *Medical Education in the United States and Canada: A Report to the Carnegie Foundation for the Advancement of Teaching* (New York: Carnegie Foundation, 1910).

24. P. Starr, *The Social Transformation of American Medicine* (New York: Basic Books, 1982).

25. Flexner, *Medical Education*; Starr, *Social Transformation of American Medicine.*

26. C. G. Jung, *Man and His Symbols* (Garden City, NY: Doubleday, 1964); Greek Mythology.com, "Icarus," accessed June 17, 2024, https://www.greekmythology.com /Myths/Mortals/Icarus/icarus.html.

27. Jung, *Man and His Symbols.*

28. Luke 4:23 (King James Version).

Appendix B

1. American Academy of Family Physicians, *Palliative and End-of-Life Care*, Recommended Curriculum Guidelines for Family Medicine Residents, AAFP repr. no. 269 (American Academy of Family Physicians, September 2020), https://www.aafp.org/dam /AAFP/documents/medical_education_residency/program_directors/Reprint269_Pal liative.pdf; R. B. Cutler, D. A. Fishbain, H. L. Rosomoff, E. Abdel-Moty, T. M. Khalil, and R. S. Rosomoff, "Does Nonsurgical Pain Center Treatment of Chronic Pain Return Patients to Work? A Review and Meta-Analysis of the Literature," *Spine* 19, no. 6 (March 15, 1994): 643–52, https://doi.org/10.1097/00007632-199403001-00002; L. Freilich, J. S. Lyles, M. Sharma, S. Kavuturu, H. S. Laird-Fick, K. Grayson-Sneed, and R. C. Smith, "A Curriculum for Training Medical Faculty to Teach Mental Health Care—and Their Responses to the Learning," *Journal of Clinical Outcomes Management* 27, no. 4 (July 2020): 166–73, https://doi.org/10.12788/jcom.0016; K. A. Grayson-Sneed, F. C. Dwamena, S. Smith, H. S. Laird-Fick, L. Freilich, and R. C. Smith, "A Questionnaire Identifying Four Key Components of Patient Satisfaction with Physician Communica-

tion," *Patient Education and Counseling* 99, no. 6 (June 2016): 1054–61, https://doi
.org/10.1016/j.pec.2016.01.002; K. A. Grayson-Sneed and R. C. Smith, "A Research
Coding Method to Evaluate a Smoking Cessation Model for Training Residents—A Preliminary Report," *Patient Education and Counseling* 101, no. 3 (March 2018): 541–45,
https://doi.org/10.1016/j.pec.2017.09.010; K. A. Grayson-Sneed and R. C. Smith,
"A Research Coding Method to Evaluate Medical Clinicians Conduct of Behavioral
Health Care in Patients with Unexplained Symptoms," *Patient Education and Counsel-
ing* 101, no. 4 (April 2018): 743–49, https://doi.org/10.1016/j.pec.2017.10.006; K. A.
Grayson-Sneed, S. W. Smith, and R. C. Smith, "A Research Coding Method for the Basic
Patient-Centered Interview," *Patient Education and Counseling* 100, no. 3 (March 2017):
518–25, https://doi.org/10.1016/j.pec.2016.10.003; L. A. Green, S. M. Jones, G. Fetter
Jr., and P. A. Pugno, "Preparing the Personal Physician for Practice: Changing Family
Medicine Residency Training to Enable New Model Practice," *Academic Medicine* 82,
no. 12 (December 2007): 1220–27, https://doi.org/10.1097/ACM.0b013e318159d070;
T. M. Kashner, K. Rost, B. Cohen, M. Anderson, and G. R. Smith Jr., "Enhancing the
Health of Somatization Disorder Patients: Effectiveness of Short-Term Group Therapy,"
Psychosomatics 36, no. 5 (September–October 1995): 462–70, https://doi.org/10.1016
/S0033-3182(95)71627-9; W. Katon, M. Von Korff, E. Lin, E. Walker, G. E. Simon,
T. Bush, P. Robinson, and J. Russo, "Collaborative Management to Achieve Treat-
ment Guidelines: Impact on Depression in Primary Care," *JAMA* 273, no. 1 (April
5, 1995): 1026–31, https://doi.org/10.1001/jama.1995.03520370068039; I. Klimes,
R. A. Mayou, M. J. Pearce, L. Coles, and J. R. Fagg, "Psychological Treatment for
Atypical Non-Cardiac Chest Pain: A Controlled Evaluation," *Psychological Medicine* 20,
no. 3 (August 1990): 605–11, https://doi.org/10.1017/s0033291700017116; R. M.
Leipzig, L. Granville, D. Simpson, M. B. Anderson, K. Sauvigné, and R. P. Soriano,
"Keeping Granny Safe on July 1: A Consensus on Minimum Geriatrics Competencies
for Graduating Medical Students," *Academic Medicine* 84, no. 5 (May 2009): 604–10,
https://doi.org/10.1097/ACM.0b013e31819fab70; J. S. Lyles, A. Hodges, C. Collins,
C. Lein, C. W. Given, B. Given, D. D'Mello et al., "Using Nurse Practitioners to
Implement an Intervention in Primary Care for High-Utilizing Patients with Medically
Unexplained Symptoms," *General Hospital Psychiatry* 25, no. 2 (March–April 2003):
63–73, https://doi.org/10.1016/s0163-8343(02)00288-8; L. Mezei, B. B. Murinson,
and Johns Hopkins Pain Curriculum Development Team, "Pain Education in North
American Medical Schools," *Journal of Pain* 12, no. 12 (December 2011): 1199–1208,
https://doi.org/10.1016/j.jpain.2011.06.006; J. Peters, R. G. Large, and G. Elkind,
"Follow-Up Results from a Randomised Controlled Trial Evaluating In- and Outpatient Pain Management Programmes," *Pain* 50, no. 1 (July 1992): 41–50, https://doi
.org/10.1016/0304-3959(92)90110-W; K. Rost, T. M. Kashner, and R. G. Smith Jr.,
"Effectiveness of Psychiatric Intervention with Somatization Disorder Patients: Improved
Outcomes at Reduced Costs," *General Hospital Psychiatry* 16, no. 6 (November 1994):
381–87, https://doi.org/10.1016/0163-8343(94)90113-9; M. Sharpe, R. Peveler, and
R. Mayou, "The Psychological Treatment of Patients with Functional Somatic Symptoms: A Practical Guide," *Journal of Psychosomatic Research* 36, no. 6 (September 1992):
515–29, https://doi.org/10.1016/0022-3999(92)90037-3; G. R. Smith Jr., K. Rost, and
T. M. Kashner, "A Trial of the Effect of a Standardized Psychiatric Consultation on

Health Outcomes and Costs in Somatizing Patients," *Archives of General Psychiatry* 52, no. 3 (March 1995): 238–43, https://doi.org/10.1001/archpsyc.1995.03950150070012; R. C. Smith, H. Laird-Fick, D. D'Mello, F. C. Dwamena, A. Romain, J. Olson, K. Kent et al., "Addressing Mental Health Issues in Primary Care: An Initial Curriculum for Medical Residents," *Patient Education and Counseling* 94, no. 1 (January 2014): 33–42, https://doi.org/10.1016/j.pec.2013.09.010; R. C. Smith, H. Laird-Fick, F. C. Dwamena, L. Freilich, B. Mavis, K. Grayson-Sneed, D. D'Mello, M. Spoolstra, and D. Solomon, "Teaching Residents Mental Health Care," *Patient Education and Counseling* 101, no. 12 (December 2018): 2145–55, https://doi.org/10.1016/j.pec.2018.07.023; H. M. Warwick, D. M. Clark, A. M. Cobb, and P. M. Salkovskis, "A Controlled Trial of Cognitive-Behavioural Treatment of Hypochondriasis," *British Journal of Psychiatry* 169, no. 2 (August 1996): 189–95, https://doi.org/10.1192/bjp.169.2.189.

2. A. H. Fortin VI, F. C. Dwamena, R. M. Frankel, B. L. Lepisto, and R. C. Smith, *Smith's Patient-Centered Interviewing: An Evidence-Based Method*, 4th ed. (New York: McGraw-Hill Education, 2018); R. C. Smith, D. D'Mello, G. G. Osborn, L. Freilich, F. C. Dwamena, and H. Laird-Fick, *Essentials of Psychiatry in Primary Care: Behavioral Health in the Medical Setting* (New York: McGraw-Hill Education, 2019).

3. Smith, D'Mello, Osborn et al., *Essentials of Psychiatry*.

4. Smith, D'Mello, Osborn et al., *Essentials of Psychiatry*.

5. American Academy of Family Physicians, *Palliative and End-of-Life*; A. J. Barsky and G. L. Klerman, "Overview: Hypochondriasis, Bodily Complaints, and Somatic Styles," *American Journal of Psychiatry* 140, no. 3 (March 1983): 273–83, https://doi .org/10.1176/ajp.140.3.273; Cutler et al., "Nonsurgical Pain Center Treatment"; F. V. deGruy 3rd, "A Note on the Partnership between Psychiatry and Primary Care," *American Journal of Psychiatry* 163, no. 9 (September 2006): 1487–89, https://doi .org/10.1176/ajp.2006.163.9.1487; Green et al., "Preparing the Personal Physician"; Kashner et al., "Enhancing the Health"; W. Katon, P. Robinson, M. Von Korff, E. Lin, T. Bush, E. Ludman, G. Simon, and E. Walker, "A Multifaceted Intervention to Improve Treatment of Depression in Primary Care," *Archives of General Psychiatry* 53, no. 10 (October 1996): 924–32, https://doi.org/10.1001/archpsyc.1996.01830100072009; W. Katon, J. Russo, M. Von Korff, E. Lin, G. Simon, T. Bush, E. Ludman, and E. Walker, "Long-Term Effects of a Collaborative Care Intervention in Persistently Depressed Primary Care Patients," *Journal of General Internal Medicine* 17, no. 10 (October 2002): 741–48, https://doi.org/10.1046/j.1525-1497.2002.11051.x; W. Katon, M. Von Korff, E. Lin, T. Bush, J. Russo, P. Lipscomb, and E. Wagner, "A Randomized Trial of Psychiatric Consultation with Distressed High Utilizers," *General Hospital Psychiatry* 14, no. 2 (March 1992): 86–98, https://doi.org/10.1016/0163-8343(92)90033-7; W. Katon, M. Von Korff, E. Lin, and G. Simon, "Rethinking Practitioner Roles in Chronic Illness: The Specialist, Primary Care Physician, and the Practice Nurse," *General Hospital Psychiatry* 23, no. 3 (2001): 138–44, https://doi.org/10.1016/S0163 -8343(01)00136-0; W. Katon, M. Von Korff, E. Lin, G. Simon, E. Walker, J. Unützer, T. Bush, J. Russo, and E. Ludman, "Stepped Collaborative Care for Primary Care Patients with Persistent Symptoms of Depression: A Randomized Trial," *Archives of General Psychiatry* 56, no. 12 (December 1999): 1109–15, https://doi.org/10.1001 /archpsyc.56.12.1109; Katon, Von Korff, Lin, Walker et al., "Collaborative Manage-

ment"; Klimes et al., "Psychological Treatment"; K. Kroenke and R. L. Spitzer, "The PHQ-9: A New Depression Diagnostic and Severity Measure," *Psychiatric Annals* 32, no. 9 (September 2002): 509–15, https://doi.org/10.3928/0048-5713-20020901-06; Leipzig et al., "Keeping Granny Safe"; Mezei, Murinson, and Johns Hopkins Pain Curriculum Development Team, "Pain Education"; Peters, Large, and Elkind, "Follow-Up Results"; B. L. Rollman, B. H. Belnap, S. Mazumdar, P. R. Houck, F. Zhu, W. Gardner, C. F. Reynolds 3rd, H. C. Schulberg, and M. K. Shear, "A Randomized Trial to Improve the Quality of Treatment for Panic and Generalized Anxiety Disorders in Primary Care," *Archives of General Psychiatry* 62, no. 12 (December 2005): 1332–41, https://doi.org/10.1001/archpsyc.62.12.1332; Rost, Kashner, and Smith, "Effectiveness of Psychiatric Intervention"; Sharpe, Peveler, and Mayou, "Psychological Treatment of Patients"; Smith, Rost, and Kashner, "Trial of the Effect"; Smith, Laird-Fick, D'Mello et al., "Addressing Mental Health Issues"; M. D. Sullivan, S. A. Cole, G. E. Gordon, S. R. Hahn, and R. G. Kathol, "Psychiatric Training in Medicine Residencies: Current Needs, Practices, and Satisfaction," *General Hospital Psychiatry* 18, no. 2 (March 1996): 95–101, https://doi.org/10.1016/0163-8343(95)00129-8; Warwick et al., "Controlled Trial."

6. Grayson-Sneed, Dwamena et al., "Questionnaire"; Grayson-Sneed and Smith, "Research Coding Method to Evaluate Smoking Cessation"; Grayson-Sneed and Smith, "Research Coding Method to Evaluate Medical Clinicians"; Grayson-Sneed, Smith, and Smith, "Research Coding Method for Patient-Centered Interview"; Lyles, Hodges et al., "Using Nurse Practitioners"; Smith, D'Mello, Osborn et al., *Essentials of Psychiatry*; R. C. Smith, J. C. Gardiner, Z. Luo, S. Schooley, L. Lamerato, and K. Rost, "Primary Care Physicians Treat Somatization," *Journal of General Internal Medicine* 24, no. 7 (July 2009): 829–32, https://doi.org/10.1007/s11606-009-0992-y; Smith, Laird-Fick, D'Mello et al., "Addressing Mental Health Issues"; Smith, Laird-Fick, Dwamena et al., "Teaching Residents Mental Health Care"; R. C. Smith, J. S. Lyles, J. C. Gardiner, C. Sirbu, A. Hodges, C. Collins, F. C. Dwamena et al., "Primary Care Clinicians Treat Patients with Medically Unexplained Symptoms: A Randomized Controlled Trial," *Journal of General Internal Medicine* 21, no. 7 (July 2006): 671–77, https://doi .org/10.1111/j.1525-1497.2006.00460.x.

7. Smith, Laird-Fick, Dwamena et al., "Teaching Residents Mental Health Care."

8. Smith, D'Mello, Osborn et al., *Essentials of Psychiatry*.

9. R. A. Orfaly, J. C. Frances, P. Campbell, B. Whittemore, B. Joly, and H. Koh, "Train-the-Trainer as an Educational Model in Public Health Preparedness," *Journal of Public Health Management and Practice* 11, no. 6 (November 2005): S123–27, https://doi.org/10.1097/00124784-200511001-00021; K. Skeff, "Successful Models of Faculty Development Train-the-Trainer Model," in *Models That Work: The Nuts and Bolts of Faculty Development for General Internal Medicine, Family Medicine, and General Pediatrics Conference*, 49–54, 142–45 (Orlando, FL: US Department of Health and Human Services, Health Resources and Services Administration, and the Ambulatory Pediatric Association, 1998).

10. E. J. Hahn, M. P. Noland, M. K. Rayens, and D. M. Christie, "Efficacy of Training and Fidelity of Implementation of the Life Skills Training Program," *Journal of School Health* 72, no. 7 (September 2002): 282–87, https://doi.org/10.1111/j.1746-1561.2002 .tb01333.x; P. J. Hinds, M. Patterson, and J. Pfeffer, "Bothered by Abstraction: The

Effect of Expertise on Knowledge Transfer and Subsequent Novice Performance," *Journal of Applied Psychology* 86, no. 6 (December 2001): 1232–43, https://doi.org /10.1037/0021-9010.86.6.1232; Orfaly et al., "Train-the-Trainer."

11. Freilich et al., "Curriculum for Training"; Lyles, Hodges et al., "Using Nurse Practitioners"; Smith, Laird-Fick, D'Mello et al., "Addressing Mental Health Issues"; Smith, Laird-Fick, Dwamena et al., "Teaching Residents Mental Health Care."

12. Freilich et al., "Curriculum for Training."

13. M. Ansseau, M. Dierick, F. Buntinkx, P. Cnockaert, J. De Smedt, M. Van Den Haute, and D. Vander Mijnsbrugge, "High Prevalence of Mental Disorders in Primary Care," *Journal of Affective Disorders* 78, no. 1 (January 2004): 49–55, https://doi.org/10.1016/s0165-0327(02)00219-7; K. Kroenke, "The Interface between Physical and Psychological Symptoms," *Primary Care Companion Journal of Clinical Psychiatry* 5, suppl. 7 (2003): 11–18, https://www.psychiatrist.com/wp-content/up loads/2021/02/24910_interface-between-physical-psychological-symptoms.pdf; Smith, D'Mello, Osborn et al., *Essentials of Psychiatry.*

14. Association of American Medical Colleges, "Table 1: US Medical School Faculty by Department, 2021," 2023, https://www.aamc.org/download/494988/data/18table1 .pdf; Wikipedia, "List of Medical Schools in the United States," updated June 4, 2024, https://en.wikipedia.org/wiki/List_of_medical_schools_in_the_United_States.

15. Association of American Medical Colleges, "Table 1."

16. B. J. Burns, J. E. Scott, J. D. Burke Jr., and L. G. Kessler, "Mental Health Train- ing of Primary Care Residents: A Review of Recent Literature (1974–1981)," *General Hospital Psychiatry* 5, no. 3 (September 1983): 157–69, https://doi.org/10.1016/0163 -8343(83)90051-8; A. Chur-Hansen, J. E. Carr, C. Bundy, J. J. Sanchez-Sosa, S. Tapa- nya, and S. H. Wahass, "An International Perspective on Behavioral Science Education in Medical Schools," *Journal of Clinical Psychology in Medical Settings* 15, no. 1 (March 2008): 45–53, https://doi.org/10.1007/s10880-008-9092-0; P. A. Cuff and N. A. Vanselow (eds.), *Improving Medical Education: Enhancing the Behavioral and Social Sci- ence Content of Medical School Curricula* (Washington, DC: National Academies Press, 2004);S. Melek and D. Norris, *Chronic Conditions and Comorbid Psychological Disorders*, Milliman Research Report (Seattle, WA: Milliman, July 2008), https://www.cbhc.org /wp-content/uploads/2015/11/chronic-conditions-and-comorbid-RR07-01-08.pdf.

17. Freilich et al., "Curriculum for Training"; Lyles, Hodges et al., "Using Nurse Practitioners"; Smith, Laird-Fick, D'Mello et al., "Addressing Mental Health Issues"; Smith, Laird-Fick, Dwamena et al., "Teaching Residents Mental Health Care."

18. S. E. Skochelak and S. J. Stack, "Creating the Medical Schools of the Fu- ture," *Academic Medicine* 92, no. 1 (January 2017): 16–19, https://doi.org/10.1097 /ACM.0000000000001160.

19. R. C. Brownson, G. A. Colditz, and E. K. Proctor (eds.), *Dissemination and Implementation Research in Health: Translating Science to Practice* (Oxford, UK: Oxford University Press, 2012), 28; A. B. Hamilton, A. N. Cohen, and A. S. Young, "Organiza- tional Readiness in Specialty Mental Health Care," *Journal of General Internal Medicine* 25, supp. 1 (January 2010): 27–31, https://doi.org/10.1007/s11606-009-1133-3; H. I. Meissner, R. E. Glasgow, C. A. Vinson, D. Chambers, R. C. Brownson, L. W. Green, A. S. Ammerman, B. J. Weiner, and B. Mittman, "The US Training Institute for Dis-

semination and Implementation Research in Health," *Implementation Science* 8 (January 24, 2013): 12, https://doi.org/10.1186/1748-5908-8-12; P. Mendel, L. S. Meredith, M. Schoenbaum, C. D. Sherbourne, and K. B. Wells, "Interventions in Organizational and Community Context: A Framework for Building Evidence on Dissemination and Implementation in Health Services Research," *Administration and Policy in Mental Health* 35, nos. 1–2 (March 2008): 21–37, https://doi.org/10.1007/s10488-007-0144 -9; E. K. Proctor, J. Landsverk, G. Aarons, D. Chambers, C. Glisson, and B. Mittman, "Implementation Research in Mental Health Services: An Emerging Science with Conceptual, Methodological, and Training Challenges," *Administration and Policy in Mental Health* 36, no. 1 (January 2009): 24–34, https://doi.org/10.1007/s10488-008-0197-4; B. J. Weiner, H. Amick, and S.-Y. D. Lee, "Conceptualization and Measurement of Organizational Readiness for Change: A Review of the Literature in Health Services Research and Other Fields," *Medical Care Research and Review* 65, no. 4 (August 2008): 379–436, https://doi.org/10.1177/1077558708317802.

20. J. W. Dearing and K. Kee, "Historical Roots of Dissemination and Implementation Science," in *Dissemination and Implementation Research in Health: Translating Science to Practice*, ed. R. C. Brownson, G. A. Colditz, and E. K. Proctor, 55–71 (Oxford, UK: Oxford University Press, 2012); E. M. Rogers, *Diffusion of Innovations*, 5th ed. (New York: Free Press, 2003).

21. Dearing and Kee, "Historical Roots of Dissemination"; Rogers, *Diffusion of Innovations*.

22. A. L. Greer, "The State of the Art versus the State of the Science: The Diffusion of New Medical Technologies into Practice," *International Journal of Technology Assessment in Health Care* 4, no. 1 (January 1988): 5–26, https://doi.org/10.1017/s02664623 00003202; Rogers, *Diffusion of Innovations*.

23. Rogers, *Diffusion of Innovations*.

24. D. M. Berwick, "Disseminating Innovations in Health Care," *JAMA* 289, no. 15 (April 16, 2003): 1969–75, https://doi.org/10.1001/jama.289.15.1969; Rogers, *Diffusion of Innovations*.

25. Rogers, *Diffusion of Innovations*.

26. Rogers, *Diffusion of Innovations*.

27. J. W. Dearing and M. W. Kreuter, "Designing for Diffusion: How Can We Increase Uptake of Cancer Communication Innovations?" *Patient Education and Counseling* 81, suppl. (December 2010): S100–10, https://doi.org/10.1016/j.pec.2010.10.013.

28. Hamilton, Cohen, and Young, "Organizational Readiness"; W. E. K. Lehman, J. M. Greener, and D. D. Simpson, "Assessing Organizational Readiness for Change," *Journal of Substance Abuse Treatment* 22, no. 4 (June 2002): 197–209, https://doi .org/10.1016/s0740-5472(02)00233-7.

29. American Academy of Family Physicians, *Palliative and End-of-Life*; Cutler et al., "Nonsurgical Pain Center Treatment"; Green et al., "Preparing the Personal Physician"; Kashner et al., "Enhancing the Health"; Katon, von Korff, Lin, Walker et al., "Collaborative Management"; Klimes et al., "Psychological Treatment"; Leipzig et al., "Keeping Granny Safe"; Mezei, Murinson, and Johns Hopkins Pain Curriculum Development Team, "Pain Education"; Peters, Large, and Elkind, "Follow-Up Results"; Rost, Kashner, and Smith, "Effectiveness of Psychiatric Intervention"; Sharpe, Peveler, and Mayou,

"Psychological Treatment of Patients"; Smith, Rost, and Kashner, "Trial of the Effect"; Smith, Gardiner, Luo et al., "Primary Care Physicians Treat Somatization"; Smith, Laird-Fick, D'Mello et al., "Addressing Mental Health Issues"; Smith, Lyles, Gardiner et al., "Primary Care Clinicians Treat Patients"; Warwick et al., "Controlled Trial."

30. D. E. Kern, P. A. Thomas, and M. T. Hughes (eds.), *Curriculum Development for Medical Education: A Six-Step Approach* (Baltimore, MD: Johns Hopkins University Press, 2009).

31. T. F. Bishop, J. K. Seirup, H. A. Pincus, and J. S. Ross, "Population of US Practicing Psychiatrists Declined, 2003–13, Which May Help Explain Poor Access to Mental Health Care," *Health Affairs* 35, no. 7 (July 1, 2016): 1271–77, https://doi.org/10.1377/hlthaff.2015.1643; B. Burns et al., "Mental Health Training"; Cuff and Vanselow, *Improving Medical Education.*

32. A. Naess, *Ecology of Wisdom* (London: Penguin Classics, 2016).

33. Kaiser Family Foundation, "Total Number of Medical School Graduates," accessed June 17, 2024, https://www.kff.org/other/state-indicator/total-medical-school-graduates/?currentTimeframe=0&sortModel=%7B%22colId%22:%22Location%22,%22sort%22:%22asc%22%7D.

34. American Association of Nurse Practitioners, "Planning Your Nurse Practitioner (NP) Education," accessed June 17, 2024, https://www.aanp.org/student-resources/planning-your-np-education#:~:text=Select%20Your%20NP%20Program,the%20perfect%20program%20for%20you%3F; ARC-PA, "Entry Level Accredited Programs," accessed June 17, 2024, http://www.arc-pa.org/accreditation/accredited-programs/; PhysicianAssistantEDU.org, "Physician Assistant Schools," accessed June 17, 2024, https://www.physicianassistantedu.org/how-to-become; E. S. Salsberg, "Changes in the Pipeline of New NPs and RNs: Implications for Health Care Delivery and Educational Capacity," *Health Affairs*, June 5, 2018, https://doi.org/10.1377/forefront.20180524.993081.

35. M. Seybold, "The Apocryphal Twain: 'The Things You Didn't Do,'" Center for Mark Twain Studies, June 28, 2019, https://marktwainstudies.com/the-apocryphal-twain-the-things-you-didnt-do/.

36. D. M. Berwick and J. A. Finkelstein, "Preparing Medical Students for the Continual Improvement of Health and Health Care: Abraham Flexner and the New 'Public Interest,'" *Academic Medicine* 85, suppl. 9 (September 2010): S56–65, https://doi.org/10.1097/ACM.0b013e3181ead779.

37. Z. Luo, J. C. Gardiner, and R. C. Smith, "Costs of a Train-the-Trainer Program to Teach Primary Care Faculty Mental Health Care," *Medical Care* 59, no. 11 (November 2021): 970–74, https://doi.org/10.1097/MLR.0000000000001621.

38. S. P. Melek, D. T. Norris, and J. Paulus, *Economic Impact of Integrated Medical-Behavioral Healthcare: Implications for Psychiatry*, Milliman American Psychiatric Association Report (Denver, CO: Milliman, April 2014), https://www.coloradocoalition.org/sites/default/files/2017-01/milliaman-apa-economicimpactofintegratedmedicalbehavioralhealthcare2014.pdf.

Appendix C

1. J. Kania, M. Kramer, and P. Senge, *The Water of Systems Change* (Boston: Financial Services Group, June 2018), https://www.fsg.org/publications/water_of_systems_change.

2. R. Pearl, *Mistreated: Why We Think We're Getting Good Health Care—and Why We're Usually Wrong* (New York: PublicAffairs, 2017); R. Pearl, *Uncaring: How the Culture of Medicine Kills Doctors and Patients* (New York: PublicAffairs, 2021).

3. D. M. Berwick, "Moral Choices for Today's Physician," *JAMA* 318, no. 21 (December 5, 2017): 2081–82, https://doi.org/10.1001/jama.2017.16254; D. M. Berwick, "The Moral Determinants of Health," *JAMA* 324, no. 3 (July 21, 2020): 225–26, https://doi.org/10.1001/jama.2020.11129.

4. Pearl, *Uncaring*.

5. F. Capra and P. Luisi, *The Systems View of Life: A Unifying Vision* (Cambridge, UK: Cambridge University Press, 2014); T. S. Kuhn, *The Structure of Scientific Revolutions* (Chicago: University of Chicago Press, 1962); P. Feyerabend, *Against Method*, 4th ed. (London: Verso, 2010); A. Naess, *Ecology of Wisdom* (London: Penguin Classics, 2016).

Index

About the Author

Robert C. Smith, MD, MACP, is a University Distinguished Professor and a professor of medicine and psychiatry emeritus at Michigan State University, East Lansing. With many publications, awards, and strong grant support, he has been involved in teaching and research in patient-centered communication and primary care mental health since 1985.

Smith and his colleagues defined the first evidence-based patient-centered interview, now published in a popular interviewing textbook, *Smith's Patient-Centered Interviewing: An Evidence-Based Method* (4th ed., 2018). It is used in medical, nursing, and other health care schools in the United States and abroad for teaching interviewing and the doctor-patient relationship.

Smith's group also identified the first evidence-based method, the mental health care model, to guide primary care clinicians in managing mental health and substance-use problems. *Essentials of Psychiatry in Primary Care: Behavioral Health in the Medical Setting* (2019) resulted and is widely used to teach primary care mental health. Visit him at https://www.robertcsmithmd.com/, https://www.linkedin.com/in/robertcsmithmd/, and https://x.com/RobertCSmithMD.

.